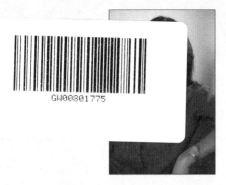

ABOUT THE AUTHOR

Belinda Neil joined the NSW Police in 1987 at the age of nineteen. During her eighteen-year police career she worked in general duties, as an undercover operative, and as a major crime squad detective investigating illicit drug operations, organised crime, and homicide. Belinda was also a police hostage negotiator and trained at the counter-terrorist level. At 32 she was a team leader for one of only five counter-terrorist negotiation teams for the Sydney 2000 Olympics. In 2002 Belinda was promoted to the rank of Inspector, one of the youngest operational inspectors in the state at that time.

In 2005 Belinda medically retired due to post-traumatic stress disorder, developed as a result of the many traumatic incidents she had attended.

One of Belinda's main aims is to raise awareness about post-traumatic stress disorder, especially after having learnt so much through research and therapy. She is also passionate about communication and negotiation. Her other interests and hobbies include public speaking, surfing, keeping fit, and riding her motorcycle.

Belinda lives south of Sydney with her two children.

UNDER SIEGE

BELINDA NEIL

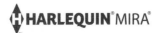

All events in this book are real, but some names, appearances, dates and locations have been changed.

First Published July 2014
Second Australian Paperback Edition 2016
ISBN 9781760374723

UNDER SIEGE
© Belinda Neil 2014

Published by
Harlequin Mira
An imprint of Harlequin Enterprises (Australia) Pty Ltd.
Level 13, 201 Elizabeth Street
SYDNEY NSW 2000
AUSTRALIA

® and TM are trademarks of Harlequin Enterprises Limited or its corporate affiliates. Trademarks indicated with ® are registered in Australia, New Zealand and in other countries.

Cover images by Newspix
Printed and bound in Australia by Griffin Press, SA

To my two beautiful children. I love you with all my heart.

*Even the healthiest individuals will become
unwell when exposed to enough trauma.*

Professor Alexander McFarlane

CONTENTS

PROLOGUE JANUARY 2004

I cannot move, I cannot run. I stare wide-eyed, my heart in my mouth, as she crawls towards me. I want to scream but no words come. What can I do? Her eyes look into mine, begging me to help. She raises one arm towards me. I watch as her blood runs down it. My breathing accelerates, fast and shallow, in and out, making me light-headed. My chest constricts, as if someone is sitting on it, and I find it difficult to breathe. I feel I am going to choke. Blood pours from the gaping wound in her neck, running down her face, pooling beneath her. Still she crawls towards me, one hand outstretched.

I am immobile, helpless.

'Can you tell me more about these images?' the psychiatrist asks.

The same girl is lying on a hospital trolley, her pale skin curling at the deep cut in her throat. Twigs and leaf litter are strewn through her hair; her stomach is smeared with faeces.

Why do I have to go through this again and again? I don't want to think about it. I don't want to see her anymore.

The psychiatrist looks at me, waiting. I want to unburden myself to him, describe the horrors that live in my mind, but I can barely speak about them. I look at the man opposite me, shake my head and mumble, 'No'. The image disappears, and I am spent. How the hell am I supposed to discuss my innermost horrors with someone I met forty minutes ago? I just want to curl up in bed and cry and cry and cry.

The psychiatrist's job was to determine whether my work had made me psychologically ill. Years as a homicide investigator and undercover operative, as well as my involvement in intense, high-risk negotiation and tactical operations, the long working hours with no time to recover from one traumatic incident before being thrown into the next, had taken their toll. I was exhausted, falling apart.

What could I do? I was a police hostage negotiator, trained to counter-terrorist-level negotiation, and an Inspector of police, and I could not even consider volunteering to work at my children's school canteen. I simply couldn't handle the pressure of taking lunch orders from schoolkids or working out their change. I could barely leave the house, and when I did I would count the moments before I could return to my sanctuary. I had been reduced to this.

Everything came to a head when I took a trip away to a day spa in the Southern Highlands about 100 kilometres south of Sydney. My mind a jumbled mess of horrifying memories, I found myself in a beautiful spot overlooking the Morton National park, so serene, so peaceful, so calm, so at odds with the confusion in my head. I wanted to be part of that vista. I wanted to feel serene and peaceful and calm.

I was on the edge. I could see no way out. I couldn't cope with work or my role as mother of two beautiful young children. I wanted relief. I had spent ten years as a police negotiator speaking to people at their lowest point, convincing them not to end their lives and now I had reached the brink: my career in the police force was over, my marriage was about to end. I was negotiating with myself to save myself.

I needed to bring myself back from the precipice. I knew I needed help.

How, I wondered, had it come to this?

CHAPTER

1

Early years

I grew up in the Sutherland Shire, in the southern suburbs of Sydney, the eldest of three children. Dad was an electrical engineer and Mum a registered nurse. I was always very independent, which my mother recognised, and I had a strong sense of adventure, which showed from an early age. On my second day at kindergarten at St Patrick's primary school, Sutherland, I told Mum I wanted to catch the bus to school on my own; she let me. When I was small we used to visit the dairy farm Mum's parents ran at Bellingen on the mid north coast of New South Wales. I quickly decided that Pop, my grandfather, had the most interesting job around the place. As a result, however hard he tried he could never sneak out of the house without me trailing behind. I got into a lot of mischief, including being kicked in the stomach and winded by a calf one day.

In 1976 Dad, who worked for the NSW Electricity Commission, was transferred to Papua New Guinea. For two and a half years we lived in a compound in Boroko, Port Moresby. The Catholic school I attended had students from all over the world, including from Cyprus, Italy and the Philippines.

When I was ten my parents let me go to Rabaul for a student exchange program/school excursion. I lived with a local family – the parents were Chinese and Japanese – for a week. The island of Rabaul above PNG has active volcanoes, and on the second last day of the trip we students went for an excursion into one of them. The smell of sulphur was incredible, and so were the pools of yellow liquid inside the volcano. We had to hold our noses as we walked around inside the crater. The next day I suffered bad headaches, was dizzy and vomiting from the effects of the gas, but I always remember that trip as a wonderful experience. I suppose we would have had to be careful, and I never felt that was dangerous at all.

We returned from PNG at the end of 1978 when I was eleven. I went to Mary Immaculate College, Sutherland, where my favourite subject was mathematics. I preferred its logical nature to English, though I did enjoy public speaking and debating. As a student I was above average, but this did not translate into street smarts. I was a bit naïve, probably because my strict Catholic upbringing meant I was not allowed out very often. I never got into trouble at school except for talking too much, though that meant I was often sent out of class.

I left secondary school in 1985 and it was time for me to choose a career. Medicine was my first choice, as I'd always had an interest in helping people. However, I didn't achieve the results I needed and instead I started a business degree, working part-time as a clerk with the NSW Electricity Commission.

One day I was driving home from the Central Coast with my boss after we had inspected a couple of power stations in the Hunter and Central Coast regions. On the highway, we saw that a car had run into the back of a utility and that its front windscreen had splintered. We could see that someone was still inside the car, so I pulled over and ran across. An old man, with blood running down his face, was sitting at the wheel. 'Help me,' he kept saying. He did not look good.

While my boss quickly organised help, I got the man out of the car and sat with him on the grassy verge next to the highway, holding his hand and telling him, 'You will be okay; the ambulance will be here soon.' Before long the police crew arrived and took over. I was impressed with the way they took control of the situation. One started directing traffic around the accident area and the other spoke with the injured man, the utility driver and the ambulance officers who had arrived on the scene.

I was so relieved when the police and ambos showed up, and I started to think that perhaps I could make a difference as a police officer or a paramedic. When I made enquiries about paramedic training, however, I discovered that it was a very difficult area to get into, with limited jobs, and so I turned my attention to the New South Wales Police. As a child some of my favourite books had been the Famous Five, Hardy Boys and Nancy Drew series – all dealing with intrepid children who solved mysteries and righted wrongs – and I had always been fascinated by investigation and forensics. Being in the police force seemed to combine adventure, excitement and being useful in the community. This, I decided, was for me.

My father was not impressed with my decision. He believed I should complete my business degree. Knowing what I know now, I probably should have listened to him – but how many independent teenage daughters take any notice of their fathers?

My grandmother knew a high-ranking federal police officer, and she put in a word on my behalf. He said I shouldn't bother to train, I should just marry a copper. It was a comment that I later learned reflected one attitude – not by any means universal – towards women police at the time.

I applied to the New South Wales Police Force and was told to do a fitness test as part of the application process. On the day I arrived at the Redfern Police Academy I was feeling very nervous. Five other applicants were fidgeting as much as I was while the instructor ran through the morning's activities. The test would include an obstacle course and a 2.5-kilometre run. He took us out of the room into the main arena and walked us through the course; a walk along a balance beam, a jump over a 1.8-metre-high wall, a short run of about 400 metres, two windows to climb through, a 2.4-metre-high wire fence to scale, an adult-sized dummy to be dragged 100 metres and a handcuff machine. This was the height of an average man and had two mechanical arms, with resistance when the arms were pulled together so the ends locked. This obstacle course had to be completed in less than three minutes and we would be weighed down with an eight-kilo gun belt. As we headed for the first wall, I wondered how I was going to get over it.

We practised first. I am 1.74 metres tall and do not possess huge strength in my upper arms. One of the male recruits went straight over, making it look easy. Maybe it wasn't as hard as it looked, I thought. When it came my turn I ran at the wall and leapt off the ground, my puny arms trying to pull my weight over. I crashed down on the wrong side of the wall. It was hopeless, even more difficult than I had thought. I wasn't the only one; two others tried and, like me, hung miserably on the wrong side. One of the successful male applicants explained the technique involved; a short run, then one foot up on the wall, grab the top of the wall and use the momentum to swing over with the other leg. One of the others made it using this technique, but I tried again and failed.

At this point stubbornness took over and I told myself *I am going to get through this*. I tried again and failed. I tried again. This time I made it and I was elated: as long as I could do this during the test I would be fine. Finally, the test came. I reviewed the technique and reminded myself that I had already succeeded. I took a long run, got one foot up on the wall and grabbed the top with my hands. Only just hanging on, I managed to get one leg over. '*Yes!*' Sheer willpower gave me the strength to drag my other leg over the wall, and then I was on the other side, *Yay!* I would later discover the bruises this effort caused.

We all passed the fitness tests except one girl who couldn't make it over the wall. Vaulting over that wall was the most difficult thing we had to do, and when I consider some of the fences I later had to negotiate while chasing suspects, it was a good test. I couldn't believe it when I heard some years later that the height of the wall had been reduced to 1.5 metres, then removed from the fitness test altogether because so many prospective police officers had been unable to climb over it. In the real world building codes do not change and fences remain the same height.

There were other tests, of course, and we all had to do a long and comprehensive interview. When I finally found out

I had passed after the interview stage I was very excited. I was accepted into the intake of 4 January 1987 with approximately 190 others.

The initial training took place at Goulburn Police Academy over three months. For the first six weeks the trainers treated us very harshly. Apparently this was an exercise in character-building and intended to prepare us for life on the streets. Punishment was physical: anyone who was late to class or caught speaking out of turn would be made to do knuckle pushups on pavers that were burning hot from the sun. We were constantly reminded that on the scale of importance we were lower than a police dog.

Our training at the academy included physical, legal studies, role-play and weapons training. I soon discovered I was an average shot with the police-issue Smith and Wesson six-shot .38-calibre pistol. This did not change throughout my career; I would usually scrape through or have to redo the required annual shooting test. My forte was obviously talking and arguing. I came second in a public speaking competition and earned the nickname 'Have-a-chat'.

The day before our graduation the excitement was building: only one more day in Goulburn! We couldn't wait to get home. Then one of the instructors, referring to the extra two weeks' training that would confirm us as constables in a year's time, said: 'You will not all return to secondary training. Some of you will be killed in action as you go about your duty as police officers.' The audience went quiet for a few moments before the general buzz and excitement of the upcoming graduation took over. Whilst his words made no impact on us at that time, they would later prove to be prophetic.

On graduation day we all felt so proud of ourselves, standing to attention on the field at Goulburn in our shiny perfectly pressed new uniforms. My family was proud of me too, and my father was now supportive, knowing this was my chosen career. It was the beginning of a new adventure, although I was sad that I would no longer be working with the friends I had made.

When I was told I would be stationed at Waverley as a probationary constable, I was devastated. I had asked for Sutherland. Waverley? I had never heard of it. I felt such a fool when I found out it was in Sydney's eastern suburbs, near Bondi Beach and a five minute-drive from Maroubra. Two classmates, Nicky and Jodie, were also probationers at Waverley. Both had blonde hair, blue eyes and were gorgeous girls both in looks and nature. Some others from our class, including Tim, a lovely Greek guy, were going to the neighbouring police stations of Paddington, Rose Bay and Bondi, so that was good too.

Each of us was given a 'buddy' for six weeks. Buddies were police officers with more than five years' service assigned to show us the ropes, to help us put into practice everything we had been taught at the academy. My buddy, Ross, was most upset that I was a woman; his last buddy, also female, had caused a lot of problems through lack of commonsense, and he was very reserved and strict with me at first. It seemed I had to prove him wrong – not a great way to start. Apparently I did: he warmed up later and I discovered that he is a great guy.

Three weeks after my arrival I arrived at work in my little red Toyota Corolla about 6.45am to start my 7am shift. Ross was already there. A message came through on the police radio: someone had been trapped in a car after an accident at the corner of Darley Road and Avoca Street, Randwick. I had just driven through that intersection. Then we heard that the person trapped was one of our own; Dana, a probationary constable from a previous intake, who had also been due to start her shift at Waverley. Ross went to the accident but told me to stay at the station, believing that the scene would be too distressing for me because I knew her. Dana was a very friendly girl with a lovely caring nature.

It wasn't long before word came back to the station that Dana had died of severe head and internal injuries. I felt numb, never having experienced death so closely before. When the tears welled up, I did my best to hide them. It didn't seem right to show my feelings when other people at the police station had known her for longer than I had, and therefore had a deeper reason to grieve. Later that day I heard on the news that a drunk driver had gone through a red light, hitting Dana's car and killing her.

Mum rang me from Coffs Harbour. She was visiting my nanna, had heard the news report and was terrified that I had been the policewoman who died in the accident. It could have been, I knew. Dana lived in the southern suburbs of Sydney like me, she drove a red car like me, she was due to start at 7am at Waverley like me. What would have happened if I had left home five minutes later? It didn't bear thinking about.

It was 3.35 on the morning of 12 October and I was on routine night patrol with my partner. It was almost the end of our shift at Waverley, and we just had to make it to 7am before heading home to bed. Suddenly the police radio sounded with two beeps: 'Urgent! All cars stand by, 10 18 in pursuit of navy Nissan Starion sedan eastbound on Oxford Street Paddington, cars to assist.' 10 18 was the Rose Bay marked sedan. Another voice: '10 12 on Oxford Street now'. 10 12 was the

Paddington marked sedan. I'm sure Tim from my academy class was working from Paddington that night.

Immediately I was wide awake and alert. The pursuit of a stolen vehicle, and it was heading straight for us! We switched on the lights and sirens and went speeding towards Bondi Junction. No sign of tiredness now, every nerve was tingling, and I was glad to be strapped in as we sped around corners.

'10 18 ... suspect vehicle has just done a U-turn and is heading westbound along Oxford Street, opposite Centennial Park.' And then: '10 12 into a pole, ambulance required, persons trapped.' Again two beeps from the police radio. 'Pursuit terminated! Cars to assist 10 18 and 10 12.'

My blood went cold. *Shit ... that's Tim's car.*

When we arrived at the scene I saw it. The patrol car was wrapped around a telegraph pole, bent into a V. I could see Tim's partner, Dave, and a new buddy, Wendy – a probationary constable straight from the Academy.

Where was Tim? I looked closely at the front of the car, through the windscreen. *Oh my God ...*

Tim, who had been driving, was now sitting close to the middle of the front console. His eyes were open but his head lolled back and blood was coursing from the top of his skull. Police cars, ambulance, fire engines, cops, ambos and firies were already there. Again, I was numb. The last thing I remember was my partner driving me away from the accident while Tim was still being taken out of the car.

Tim died in hospital from severe head, chest and spinal injuries. He had been a police officer for less than seven months. A full police funeral was held for him at the Greek Orthodox church in Kingsford. Being from the same class, I was a pallbearer, along with another girl.

I contacted Tim's mother after the funeral to return a type-writer Tim had lent me and to pay my respects. When I arrived at their home both his parents were there and his mother took me straight into the lounge room and brought out a photo album dedicated to her son. She then asked me to come and have a look at his room. I agreed, but was finding it difficult to cope with their grief and sorrow. I was only nineteen and knew nothing about this level of anguish. The knowledge of the family's pain stayed with me for many years, and Tim's death would return to haunt me.

At the time I did not realise what a devastating effect these deaths had on me. I was not counselled afterwards: the police then had no formal provision for that, and whatever help was given was directed to Tim's Paddington colleagues. Instead I did what everyone else did – I drank a lot of alcohol. One night I was out drinking until 6.30am, went home for a quick shower and was at work for a 7am shift. I was too numb to worry about being over the limit: I think I felt that, if I didn't have long to live I would make the most of what life I had. I even told my parents not to worry if I died as I was doing a job I loved. The thought never entered my head that perhaps I should look for a new career path, that perhaps this job was too dangerous. I loved the type of work I was involved with, it was exciting, challenging, and I enjoyed the camaraderie I shared with my workmates.

2

Becoming a detective

Because I worked hard I was gradually given more responsibility and even though I was only a probationary constable, I was the senior officer on many occasions. On one of these I had my first brush with a homicide.

I was working a night shift with another female probationer when I noticed a car moving erratically along Bondi Road. A man was driving with a woman passenger. I turned on lights and sirens, and the car pulled into a Caltex service station. As a standard safety measure I told the radio operator where we were. My partner and I got out of our car and approached the driver. He was a very muscular and fit man who gave his name as Joe Bloggs. I told him why he had been pulled over and asked for his driver's licence. He gave it to me and told me that he and his girlfriend had been heading home from a party. I asked him to wait a few moments while

I checked his details. As long as everything was fine with his licence, I had every intention of letting him go, provided he passed a breath test.

I returned to the police car and gave all the relevant details to the radio operator. A few minutes later he came back on and asked: 'Is the radio secure?' These words made me sit up and take note. It usually meant that the person had a criminal history or outstanding warrants.

The operator confirmed his licence details with me. The next words sent my mind spinning. 'Joe Bloggs has one outstanding warrant for murder.'

Oh shit. It was early in the morning, I was still a probationary constable and we were going to arrest this man for murder. This could get very ugly.

The radio operator asked whether I needed assistance. 'Yes, that would be nice,' I said. Immediately other police cars called in that they would head my way, which was a relief.

Now, how to approach this? The radio could provide no further information about the arrest warrant, just that there was one. I weighed up a few options with my partner then made up my mind.

I walked up to Joe, who was starting to become agitated, formally told him about the warrant and said we needed to discuss it at the police station.

'Can't we sort this out tomorrow?' he asked. I said no, because of the nature of the warrant. As his girlfriend had been drinking I offered her a lift back to the station with us, which seemed to appease him.

I was a little surprised, to say the least, that everything had gone so smoothly. I quickly advised the radio operator that all was well and we were taking two people to Waverley police station, thanking the other cars for their assistance. The other

Waverley car working that night drove past us, waited, then followed us to the police station. It was nice to know we had backup if needed.

When we arrived at Waverley I asked Joe to follow me in to the dock area inside the charge room, a secure area where we put people being charged with criminal offences. This charge room is small, approximately 3m by 3.5m, not visible to the public, and the dock is about 1 x 1.5m in size and surrounded by metal bars. With Joe safely secured in the dock, I told him he was under arrest for murder. He went berserk, yelling and shouting, banging on the side of the dock area. I was thankful that we were no longer at the service station: things would have been difficult there for sure.

I rang Homicide, who told me Joe had been in a fight outside an inner-city pub. He had punched a man who fell, hit his head on the footpath and died. I told Joe that Homicide detectives would come to interview him; at that stage I think he had resigned himself to being charged. Months later one of the Homicide police told me Joe ended up pleading guilty to manslaughter.

This was my first insight into homicide investigation, and I was thankful it had gone so well. As a result I started thinking about what the future might hold for me. My work at Waverley covered all sorts of issues: from shoplifting to car accidents, break and enters in homes and businesses, robberies, prohibited drugs, missing persons, deaths, domestic violence situations, fires. I found all these things interesting, the problem being that the more interesting the job, the more likely it was that the detectives would take over. I decided fairly early that I wanted to be a detective.

After two years I was accepted to the Waverley detectives' office, with a month's probation to see whether I was good enough to train as an investigator. I passed, and was accepted as a plainclothes investigator. I was elated.

Two months later in May 1989 Jeremy, a former detective from our office who had joined the Drug Enforcement Agency, rang and asked whether I was interested in applying for the Undercover Unit, to replace a female operative who had left. The Drug Enforcement Agency consisted of the Undercover Unit, the Support Unit and four task forces, each of which had specific responsibility for dealing with middle- to upper-level drug supply. I jumped at this opportunity to do something different, to pit my mind against drug dealers. It was a challenge and I loved a challenge!

Once again I showed how inexperienced I was. The only drug I had ever touched was alcohol, albeit in excess since the deaths of Tim and Dana two years earlier. I had never even smoked a cigarette except once at a party when I was sixteen, I had been so giddy that everyone assumed I had taken something stronger. So before my interview a friend of mine took me aside and showed me how to roll a joint and pack a bong. Thank goodness he did because the DEA Undercover Unit supervisors asked me to do exactly that.

I got the job: I don't think there were any other applicants. The detective senior sergeant in charge of Waverley tried to talk me out of it, but to me it was a very exciting career move. At the Undercover Unit I was given a false identity, driver's licence, and a car, a red Mazda. I cannot remember the model although I do remember it had a sunroof. Our office was a covert factory in the inner west of Sydney and we worked permanent afternoon shifts unless we were involved in an operation.

The criminals' activities, of course, didn't revolve around standard police shifts; many of them used licensed premises, pubs, clubs and hotels as their offices. Thus on many occasions I found myself sitting in pubs and drinking beer with the locals. The undercover nature of the work made this necessary, and management accepted this as part of the job of gathering intelligence and sometimes finding more work.

It was an interesting time for a twenty-one-year-old. Now I was living in Sydney's eastern suburbs and spending my days at the beach developing a tan while in the afternoons and evenings I went out drinking beer at various pubs in the Sydney area. I also spent considerable time at Kings Cross, Sydney's red-light district and home to various organised-crime gangs.

One controversial spot was Sweethearts café in Darlinghurst Road. In June 1989, only a few months earlier, there had been a drug-related fight there and a man had been shot and killed. Arben Benny Puta was charged with murder but later acquitted. The subsequent police investigation became the subject of corruption allegations at the Wood Royal Commission (formed in 1994 to investigate the existence and extent of corruption within the NSW Police Force).

However, I knew nothing about the police investigation. My job was to find someone at Sweethearts who would sell me cocaine. Initially I went with two other undercover operatives who were going to watch me as a safety precaution. They would be inside having a coffee. I went into the café cold, with no one to introduce me. I was apprehensive, knowing someone had been murdered in the toilets at the back, exactly where I was headed to see the dealer. My hands were clammy; I kept trying to wipe them on the skirt I was wearing, I was so worried I would be caught out, kicked out or worse.

I found the dealer and went straight up to him and said, 'Can I get a fifty?' Before I could react, he grabbed my bag off my shoulder and searched it. Fortunately I was not carrying my police ID. I finally managed to say, 'What the...?'

'You a cop?' he said.

'Nah, just want a fifty.'

After being satisfied I was not a cop he gave me a small foil of cocaine for $50.00, my 'fifty'. I turned around and walked out of the café and down the street. Finally, being out of danger, I could relax.

Over the next few weeks I bought more fifties from this café. My workmates who had given me cover had other jobs so I went by myself. Eventually my drug dealer was arrested and we were able to put together a good brief of evidence against him. He went to gaol.

One of my favourite workmates was nicknamed BP, an intelligent, good-looking blue-eyed blond guy, who could talk underwater with a mouth full of marbles. I once had to meet him at the Albury Hotel in Oxford Street, a renowned gay hangout, prior to going to another job. I arrived first and it was easy to see BP coming to meet me as the gentlemen in the crowd suddenly parted like the Red Sea to allow this good-looking young man to pass through. BP quickly grabbed me and we left the hotel; I could hardly stop laughing.

BP's mischievous nature came to the fore on a number of occasions. One time, just before he was about to buy a large quantity of drugs for a buy bust, he was wearing a listening device. After various prearranged signals, arrest teams would move in and arrest him, the drug supplier and anybody else. My role was to sit in a van nearby with a supervisor (I was still very new), and listen to BP's conversations with the dealer. I was sitting in the van when BP turned on the listening device. He was talking to one of the DEA Support Unit investigators, a guy I did not know. My ears pricked up when I heard BP ask, 'So, what do you think of our new bird Wendy?' my code name in the Undercover Unit. His reply suggested that he was unable to fully contain his sexual excitement. I nearly fell off the chair laughing, especially when they told the guy, whose name was Rob, that the listening device was on: he was most embarrassed when he realised he had been set up.

After six months at the Undercover Unit I realised it wasn't for me. Going to work purporting to be someone else no longer thrilled me. Undercover work was dangerous, required a great deal of skill and was a necessary investigative tool. I didn't, however, enjoy making up a story to gain a person's trust. It made me feel uncomfortable, and this is what I was doing every single day. Besides, I had ballooned from a size 10 to a size 14 because I had been drinking beer every night, and I didn't feel healthy. I was also having a major personality clash with one of the supervisors, who was intelligent and quick-witted but very bombastic. He would constantly belittle me in front of my peers and I couldn't understand why. No one had treated me with such contempt before.

I told the senior supervisor that I preferred the investigation and arrest phases of drug work and would like a transfer back to Waverley. He said he understood why, and said the supervisor who had been causing me problems was leaving and I should stay. I was shocked: I hadn't mentioned the real reason for my request. I chose to leave anyway and joined the DEA Support Unit, which allowed me to be involved in the investigation side as well as the occasional undercover job. The hours were better, no longer permanent afternoon shifts. I was eager for a fresh start.

One day I was running solo surveillance on the home of a suspected drug dealer in Sydney's inner west. I was trying to gather evidence, such as potential drug users coming and going and any sightings of drugs and drug paraphernalia. I wanted to get a search warrant for his home. The courts don't simply provide one every time police ask for it, and a magistrate has to be given a valid reason.

As I was sitting alone in my surveillance car I saw him come out, get into a car parked in the street and drive off. I followed him and radioed back to my colleagues at the DEA office to check the car's registration. It became clear that he was driving a stolen vehicle, and several colleagues said they were on their way to help me.

This drug dealer, whose name was Ian, was no choirboy. He had a long record of drugs and violence, including robbery and assault. He was also known as a 'runner' (a person who would run when confronted by police). I was not keen to take on a dangerous criminal by myself so the rest of the team and I decided that once backup had arrived, we would follow him until we could arrest him safely and search the car for drugs.

Ian was heading west out of Sydney on Parramatta Road, driving under the speed limit so as not to draw attention to himself in a stolen car. He didn't realise he was being followed.

He turned right onto Silverwater Road. My backup had still not arrived even though I knew they would be travelling at breakneck speed. We continued along Silverwater Road, then he took the turn into the Mulawa and Silverwater correctional centres before turning into the car park of Mulawa women's prison. I couldn't believe the cheek of it: Ian was heading straight for the prison in a stolen car! My backup was now only a few minutes away and I told my supervisor Bones, a highly experienced officer whom I respected, that if Ian got out of the vehicle I was going to arrest him.

As I drove I ran a number of possibilities through my mind and I started to worry. What would I do if he ran? He was a known runner after all. What if he ran at me, or jumped back in the car and rammed into me. What would I do if he pulled a gun or a knife?

I felt for my police ID because I wasn't wearing uniform. Check. Firearm, check. It was a small five-shot Model

36 Smith & Wesson revolver, with a one-inch barrel. The standard police-issue firearm was a six-shot, Model 10 Smith & Wesson revolver with a three-inch barrel. Many undercover police preferred the five-shot Smith & Wesson because the barrel was shorter, making the weapon lighter and more easy to conceal, even though it was less accurate. This posed another problem, as shooting was not my strong point. I should have been using the standard police issue but I preferred the smaller version. I figured that with my shooting record I would have to be very close, so Ian was actually pretty safe.

Ian parked the car and opened the door. I stopped my car at an angle behind his and drew my gun. My police ID was tucked into my jeans pocket with just the badge visible. With blood rushing through my veins and a barrage of thoughts about what could go wrong, I got out of my car, moved towards Ian pointing my gun and in my best voice I screamed, 'Police! Get out of the fucking car!'

So much for being assertive.

Ian stopped, looked at me and hesitated. My heart was racing, I wasn't sure what he was going to do. He could quite easily have a weapon on the seat next to him and I couldn't see his left hand.

He continued getting out of the car. 'Face down on the ground *now*!' I yelled.

I didn't realise that the bitumen car park was feeling the full effects of a very hot summer's day. The ground was scorching. My main concern was to make sure he didn't run. There was no way I would have fired on him, for I had no authority as I could see no weapon. However, what would happen if he ran towards me just didn't bear thinking about.

Ian got face down on the ground.

'Hands on your head,' I commanded. He obeyed.

At that point my backup came over the hill like the US cavalry. I was delighted to see them, though I was feeling pretty pleased with myself. It had been a textbook arrest. Ian was handcuffed and picked up off the ground by the other police and we searched the car. We found a small quantity of white powder, so Ian was arrested and taken to the local police station.

I couldn't resist asking Ian why he hadn't run, given his history. He looked me straight in the eye and said, 'I thought about running but when I saw you holding the gun, it was shaking so much I thought you might accidentally let a shot go and I'd end up with a bullet in the bum.' So much for me thinking I had handled that situation well.

By the time I got back to our headquarters the story of my exploits had been outrageously expanded. The boss was told that my colleagues had found Ian lying on the ground of the car park, handcuffed, while I, with one foot on the ground and the other on his back, was applying lipstick while I waited for backup.

At about this time I began working alongside Rob. Our working relationship, which became a romantic one, started off awkwardly because of what he had said to BP about me during the undercover operation. However, Rob was a very dedicated officer with a rapier wit. The fact that he was tall, dark and handsome was a nice addition. He was seven years older than me and seven years senior as a police officer. He was very romantic, at one stage sending a dozen red roses to my home anonymously. He also had a sense of humour, sending a male stripper to the office one day for my birthday, something the females in the office appreciated way more than our male counterparts.

He had some interesting surveillance techniques when working with me. He would say, 'Oh here comes the crook, quick, we'd better make like boyfriend/girlfriend,' as he threw his arms around me. This always made me smile.

It was good to be in a relationship with someone who understood my irregular working hours, the overtime and the trips away throughout the state, often staying in accommodation with male workmates. We had a common area of interest as we both worked in drug investigation and high-risk policing so we could discuss and share ideas. Later, as we gradually met and worked with the same people and knew their personalities and capabilities, we were able to give each other advice.

However, because of our budding relationship, it became obvious to both of us that working together was not a good scenario. One of us needed to consider a transfer.

In June 1991 the Tactical Response Group (TRG) and the Special Weapons and Operations Squad (SWOS) were disbanded after enquiries into the deaths of Darren Brennan, shot by a member of the TRG, and David Gundy, who had been shot by a member of SWOS. As a result the State Protection Group (SPG) Tactical Operations Unit (TOU) was formed. Their mission was to resolve high-risk incidents involving armed offenders and counter-terrorist operations.

Trained along military lines, the members of the TOU are given advanced skills and weapons beyond the scope of regular police. Rob was undergoing training with the Special Air Service (SAS) in Perth (he was a member of the Police Assault Group – PAG – or the Counter-Terrorist Unit of SWOS) and and on his return to Sydney he was invited to join the SPG TOU. This suited us both as we could not continue to work together at the DEA Support Unit. Our relationship continued to develop and three years later, in November 1993, we were married.

CHAPTER

3

Learning to negotiate

The first time I heard about the Hostage Negotiation Unit was via my flatmate Sue, who worked with me at the DEA Support Unit and had a secondary role as a police negotiator with the State Protection Group. Sue and Rob both told me that there was a vacancy at the negotiators and suggested I apply.

The aim of negotiation is the peaceful resolution of high-risk or crisis situations. A high-risk incident is one in which the gravity of the offence is taken into consideration as well as any history of violent behaviour, and there is a real possibility of injury or death to anyone involved, including the perpetrator.

Before 1972 police all over the world who had to handle hostage situations either demanded the surrender of the hostage taker or brought in the police Tactical team to affect an arrest. This changed after September 1972 when Israeli athletes were taken hostage at the Olympic Village in Munich and later killed by members of the Palestinian Black September terrorist organisation. Police agencies began to consider the idea of negotiation as a principal strategy.

Two New York Police Department officers, Lieutenant Frank Bolz and Officer Harvey Schlossberg, pioneered the use of negotiation and were the first to select and train officers specifically for it. The FBI soon followed, introducing a formal hostage negotiation training course at its training academy in Quantico, Virginia.

In 1979 the first hostage negotiation course was held in Sydney and the NSW Police Hostage Negotiation Unit was formed. Its brief was to fulfil the New South Wales police policy of 'contain and negotiate' – that is, to use force only as a last resort. By the time I applied to join in 1992, the word 'hostage' had been dropped from the title because of the increasing diversity of callouts. The high-risk incidents police negotiators were trained to respond to included hostage situations, suicide intervention, kidnapping, extortion, high-risk search warrants and dangerous arrests, particularly with firearms involved, or any other situation where a trained negotiator would be able to assist other police.

I was drawn to the idea of talking to someone in a life-threatening or high-risk situation to try to diffuse and resolve the incident. Again. It was another challenge and different to normal policing. Unlike undercover work there was no need to lie to gain trust, I was not making up stories or a character. I would be putting myself forward as a police officer and was overtly accountable as a police officer, and I preferred to be straightforward.

In October 1992 I was accepted into police negotiator training. This meant three years of theoretical and practical training, all of which was continually assessed. In the first year I was required to attend Goulburn Police Academy for a two-week live-in basic course, and this was followed up with two one-week courses over the next two years. During the three years I was given the opportunity to go on call with a Sydney metropolitan negotiation team. This gave me invaluable experience outside the limitations of a role-play situation. After the initial three years there were further training days, intended to ensure negotiators were kept up to date with modern technology and negotiation methods.

Basic training included instruction on many different aspects of being a negotiator: techniques and strategies, dealing with Stockholm syndrome (the psychological state of some hostages who become attached to their captors), psychological and psychiatric issues, developing listening and other communication skills. There were other practical issues: legal aspects, equipment for negotiation, the resources and procedures of the State Protection Group. There was information about the types of incident requiring negotiation. However, counter-terrorism was only touched on during the basic course, being considered suitable only for experienced negotiators.

The course featured many role plays as a way of putting theory into practice in a controlled environment. I found this one of the most important facets of our training. We were given realistic exercises, some of which had been actual call-outs, and we worked with experienced police negotiators who had been in these situations and could provide appropriate emotional responses.

All police negotiators worked part-time while maintaining their normal full-time duties. The only full-time negotiator was the commander, whose job was to co-ordinate all the negotiators in New South Wales. The state was divided into two areas: Sydney metropolitan and country. Metropolitan negotiators worked on a rostered on-call basis. There were six metropolitan teams, each including four trained negotiators, whose roles were decided on the basis of experience, not rank. The team leader's job was to manage the team, liaise with senior officers including the TOU and the Incident Commanders, guide and be responsible for strategy, assess intelligence, monitor the welfare of the team and prepare for team meetings – directing down time when required, organising appropriate advisers and technical assistance where needed, and carrying out record management. The primary negotiator was in charge of communicating with the subject and gathering intelligence, the secondary negotiator was to support the primary negotiator and relieve him or her if required. The fourth person on the team, the recorder, was responsible for maintaining the records and providing general support to the negotiation team, including interviewing victims or witnesses for information (not always required by police taking criminal statements), organising equipment and ensuring team security.

Each team was on call once every six weeks. This period lasted for seven days, twenty-four hours a day, while at the same time we continued our normal areas of work. On-call periods started on a Wednesday, when we would go to the commander's office at the Sydney Police Centre and pick up a pager, and finished when we returned the pager the following Wednesday. Metropolitan negotiators would help in the country if required; a plane was on standby at Sydney airport twenty-four hours a day to fly anywhere in New South Wales.

As part of our training we were asked to take part in the State Protection Support Unit (SPSU) operator's course. SPSU officers worked mainly in country/regional areas (although there was a metropolitan team). Their job was to contain emergencies including sieges, suicide intervention and hostage situations with, and in some cases instead of, the TOU. As negotiators and tactical operators work together, it was advantageous to have an understanding of how the other team worked.

I undertook this course in 1994 with my dear friend and fellow negotiator Nicole and twenty-three burly males, all SPSU operatives. Of all the courses I did during my police career, this was the most physically demanding. It was held at Singleton army barracks north of Sydney for two weeks in December – one of the hottest months of the year – with time off for good behaviour on the weekend. Every day during training we wore heavy boots and full-length navy fire-retardant drill cotton overalls – absolutely stifling in the extremely hot and dry weather – and we carried water bottles.

We undertook some form of physical activity every day, including running and an obstacle course. This consisted of a number of ropes, various obstacles and rope bridges strung up over a pool. Getting across the rope bridge, I realised, meant using physical strength: not my strong point.

Nic went first. At only 1.57 metres tall, seventeen centimetres shorter than me, she could barely reach the guide ropes. I couldn't believe the effort she put in. She struggled but made it to the end. Just prior to reaching the final obstacle she looked at me and yelled out, 'If I can do it, you can do it,' then made the final plunge headfirst into the water. With that encouragement, I gritted my teeth and stepped out onto the bridge. I was fairly cardio fit, having just trained and run a half marathon before embarking on this adventure, although I was not very strong, so found grasping and pulling myself up difficult. By the time I had reached the end I had a few bruises and aching limbs, but I'd made it across.

One afternoon after a busy day the instructors drove us approximately ten kilometres away from the barracks and told us we were running back. In the energy-sapping heat we were still wearing our full-length overalls, boots and body armour, carrying a water bottle and an AR15 rifle that weighed 2.89 kilos unloaded. We formed lines and started the hard slog back to the barracks. Every so often the instructors would yell, 'Get down!'and we would dive to the side of the road and leopard crawl along the roadway until we were given the all clear to get up and keep going. This effectively doubled the time of our run.

This exercise was definitely a test of mind over matter. You had to concentrate intently just to keep putting one foot in front of the other. The heat was stifling, making it difficult to breathe, and we were battling a plague of flies. Nic and I were running next to each other, giving each other moral support. The few who found it too challenging were allowed to sit in the vehicle following us.

One feature of this course and the many others I have done is the camaraderie between participants, especially if the course is a difficult one. Nic and I, the only two girls, had developed a close mateship with many of the guys purely because we were all thrown together and had to perform the same, often very demanding, tasks. A couple of the guys offered to carry our rifles along with their own, however, they were struggling too and we wouldn't do it to them. Besides, we are both very stubborn and we needed to do it for ourselves. We did appreciate the offer.

When we finally saw the front gates to the barracks after a couple of hours, we all sighed with relief. Then it started to rain, which had a lovely cooling effect and stopped the flies for a short while. We ran into the barracks and finally the instructors told us to stop. We stopped. They told us to turn around. We turned around. They told us to start running back out. We were incredulous, surely not, but away we went again. After about ten metres they told us they were just kidding and we could stop. Mind games are not particularly amusing when you are physically exhausted.

The course included advanced weapons training with the Remington 870 pump-action shotgun and the Colt AR15/ M16 semi-automatic rifle, standard weapons for these specialised units; weaponless control including unarmed combat and use of batons (this lesson was particularly painful); and bushcraft navigation, which also meant camouflage and concealment. We were also taught close quarter battle (CQB) or armed combat inside suspect premises – houses, planes, boats, etc. The principles were speed, surprise, momentum, controlled aggression, teamwork and communication. We learned the principles of marksmanship – the ability to fire accurately and safely at close range and at long distance – methods of entry including the use of necessary tools such as window reamers, sledgehammers, rams and hydraulic tools, and how to handle exposure to chemical agents, particularly CS gas, commonly known as tear gas.

We carried out this last exercise on another stifling day in a paddock at Singleton. We were all dressed in the usual kit, full-length fire retardant overalls, as well as body armour and a gas mask. One of our instructors came up and shouted, 'Two lines, now! Let's go!' We followed him at a slow jog, sweating profusely.

Meanwhile the instructors were busy preparing saturation levels of CS gas in a hut about three metres by five metres in diameter. We were to enter the hut, be exposed to the chemical agents and learn how to use an M17 respirator gas mask, all without panicking. The instructor divided us into groups of four, with Nic and myself in the same group, the second to go in. When the first group came out ripping their gas masks off, they looked a mess, with mucus streaming from their noses, and red eyes.

'Good luck,' I said to Nic before the instructor yelled, 'Masks on!' and we went into the hut. My vision was restricted by the gas mask though I could see it was very cloudy, like a smoke haze. Then, one of the instructors, also wearing a gas mask, said, 'Masks off.' Almost immediately I had a strong chemical taste in my mouth and the back of my throat and my eyes were stinging, beginning to water as I struggled to keep them open.

The instructor came next to me and said, 'Name?'

'Belinda Neil,' I replied, attempting to hold my breath and avoid breathing the gas-contaminated air.

'Registered number?'

'23451.' *Concentrate on his voice, concentrate on his voice*, I kept saying to myself. It was almost impossible: I was getting more and more disoriented as my body gasped for oxygen. I could feel my neck and my face around my nose starting to burn: the gas was settling on my skin. Now I realised why we had been told to run beforehand – so the pores in our skin would be open ...

I was sweaty and tired and wanted more than anything to run towards the door. Only pride and downright stubbornness were keeping me there, answering the instructor's questions. In the end survival instinct took over and I had to breathe. I could feel the stinging and burning of the gas down my throat and in my eyes.

After ten or fifteen minutes he said, 'Gas, gas, gas,' which meant the conversation was over. I put the gas mask back over my head and cleared it by placing my hands over the outpiece, blowing hard. Then I gave him the thumbs-up signal to indicate I was comfortably breathing again, although all areas of my exposed skin were stinging, and I was allowed to leave the gas hut.

Outside I pulled off the mask and grabbed at my overalls pocket for a tissue because I could feel mucus running down my face. It felt like sandpaper against my irritated skin, effectively only making matters worse. Nic was bent over with contaminated nasal secretions hanging down to her knees. This was not one of our most glamorous days. Breathing in that gas sure beat inhaling Vicks VapoRub as a way of curing sinus problems.

Nic and I were determined not to let the negotiators' side down, so we weren't going to pike out of anything. After the first week when we headed home for a weekend rest, I booked myself in for a massage as my body ached all over. The masseuse was horrified when he came in and saw the number of bruises all over my legs and arms from the baton training and the obstacle course. The next time I saw my masseuse, at the end of the second week, I had a lovely collage of old and new bruises ranging from yellow/black to red/blue.

One day we were training with the AR15 semi-automatic rifle. Our targets were 100 metres away. Six of us at a time were to lie down in a row and fire five shots each at our individual targets. Then we walked down to our targets to see how we had fared. My target was a clean white sheet of paper with black target circles on it. There wasn't a single bullet hole; I thought I might have managed at least a couple of shots on the outer edges. The guy on my left had seven shots in the middle of his target, the guy on the right had eight. At least I'd helped them. There was nothing wrong with my marksmanship, I thought. I just hit the wrong targets.

Apart from this debacle, I was happy with my total result from the course. I topped the academic side and Nic came top in shooting. We received glowing reports that stated we had 'performed at a very high level, setting the standard for future negotiators attending the course'. That felt very good.

CHAPTER

4

Early days in the trade

In March 1993, five months after I had finished my first course, I was asked to stand in for one of the negotiation team members and go on call. I was still working at the DEA Support Unit. This was my first time on call and I was looking forward to getting some field experience.

One evening about 7.30 I had just finished some laps at the local pool when my negotiator's pager activated. The duty operations inspector, who co-ordinated these callouts, told me there was a siege at a major manufacturing plant at Silverwater west of Sydney. I went to my on-call car, found the correct channel on the police radio and turned on the lights and siren. The adrenalin was already racing through my system; all my senses were fully alert. On the way to the job I wondered if Rob would be there, as he was on duty at the Tactical Operations Unit (TOU).

When I arrived at a roadblock that formed the outer perimeter and was allowed through, I was taken to one of the offices within the factory. Dennis, the commander of the negotiators, was there so I knew the situation was serious: he only attended these callouts when there was a major problem. He told me that a young employee who was upset about a work-related issue had placed a Coke can full of water near the aluminium smelting furnace. If it was dropped in there would be a chemical chain reaction, and the resulting explosion could take out the nearby M4 motorway and many surrounding buildings, homes and factories. We were standing within the potential blast zone.

We couldn't contact the suspect until the TOU operators had secured the inner perimeter, making sure that no unauthorised persons could enter or leave the area. Once the Tactical team was in position, we could go ahead.

The first consideration is always how to contact the suspect. Would it be face to face? Would we use the telephone, perhaps a karaoke system or megaphone? Because of the potential risk of a huge explosion it was decided that face-to-face conversation was far too dangerous. We would contact him via telephone.

As Dennis and I were the only negotiators present and I was a very new trainee, Dennis made the telephone call. First contact is always an information-gathering exercise. We needed to know exactly who was in the room, why the man was there, his state of mind and what he wanted, whether he was armed and how dangerous he was to himself, the police and members of the public, and how volatile the situation was. In other words, we needed information that could assist both him and the police. Initial conversations are usually very demanding and active listening skills are essential. We did not know whether the person on the other end of the phone would be distressed, angry or upset.

While Dennis was on the telephone, I was busy making notes of his side of the conversation. These I knew would be required if any criminal charges were laid, and they could be subpoenaed for a court case or, at worst, a coroner's inquest. Graham our team leader had now arrived, as well as the rest of the team. However, because Dennis was on the phone building a rapport with the suspect, he remained the primary negotiator.

The large Pantech negotiators' van arrived, and we could set ourselves up properly. The truck contained two sound-proofed rooms. The first, which had a number of telephone headsets, was where the primary and secondary negotiators would be seated. The team leader, who also had a headset so he could monitor what was going on, was in the second room, watching the first through a clear partition. He had access to a phone, fax machine, and police radios. Access to this negotiators' area was very restricted, only allowed to team members, the psychiatrist who gave advice about strategy and the tactical commander.

During the evening I learned that Rob was lying in a ditch guarding the inner perimeter; conditions for the TOU guys were never as pleasant as ours. It was now raining and they were getting drenched, while remaining very warm in full fireproof overalls and body armour, their full counter-terrorist kit. The temperature within the foundry was radiating out a very unpleasant 50 degrees Celsius. Although the atmosphere within the negotiators' truck was tense we, at least, had some comforts. Though we were still within the blast zone we were enjoying cups of hot tea and coffee and eating takeaway food.

The siege went on and on. During the night, Dennis spoke to the suspect often. He was a young man who believed the company had wronged him: he even had a Eureka Stockade flag as an emblem of his preparedness to stand and fight until justice prevailed. At various times his attitude changed from hostility, threatening to blow up the factory, to frustration at his perceived injustice. As the evening wore on the threat levels changed from high to medium and back to high again. These changes and the associated adrenalin surges affected my state of alertness, and fatigue was starting to settle in. I knew I had to remain aware and ready to act if necessary: there was no room for complacency. Dennis, like the rest of us, had started work in the morning of the previous day and the siege showed no signs of ending. Graham called in a relief negotiation team to take over from us in the morning.

At this stage another problem became apparent. The M4 motorway, the main arterial roadway leading into Sydney, had been closed because it was in the blast zone and its closure was causing major chaos for morning peak-hour traffic. We were under pressure to open it again, however, we could not because the situation was too dangerous for the Tactical team to move in and make an arrest.

In the morning the relief team arrived. I felt exhausted, pleased and frustrated: exhausted from trying to take everything in, pleased that everything had worked out so far and nobody had been hurt, and frustrated because we had to hand over to another negotiating team without finishing the job ourselves.

Dennis was on the phone again, and it looked as if the young man was going to surrender. It was decided that the primary negotiator of the relief team would go forward with the TOU police on the inner perimeter and greet the young man when he gave himself up. And that's what happened. The siege ended peacefully.

I knew this was exactly what I wanted to do: work with such a well coordinated team in a challenging and potentially difficult situation. I was sure I had found the right career for me.

Four months later I was involved in a very different case. On a very cold winter evening we were called out to deal with a nineteen-year-old guy who wanted to jump off the roof of a six-storey business block near Bankstown west of Sydney. We spoke to him for about five hours, but he would not say why he had decided to commit suicide. Meanwhile his father was confronting the commander at the base of the building, insisting on speaking to his son.

Situations like these require serious consideration, and third-person intervention is not considered lightly. Seeing a family member could cause a potential suicide victim to carry out the threat. Does a family member have the right to talk to the person at risk? Why does the family member want to be there, and what are the issues for both parties? On the other hand, if the person at risk wants to talk to a family member or friend, we also need to know why. Does the person want to commit suicide in front of them? Is the family member the cause of the problem? Is there another, safer way to hold a discussion between the two parties, perhaps when the potential suicide victim is no longer in danger?

This time the commander told the young man's father that he would not be allowed on the rooftop to speak with his son. The father became irate and insisted. The commander paused, looked him in the eye and said, 'If your son felt he could talk to you, would he be on that rooftop?'

It was a comment that cut to the heart of the matter. Later it came to light that the young man had just had an argument with his father. The young guy, who was unsure about his sexuality, was having difficulty dealing with his feelings and believed his father was homophobic. We couldn't risk the father upsetting the son further in case the son became distressed enough to jump off the roof, perhaps simply to spite his father. This proved to be the right strategy: after eight hours we were able to negotiate the son to safety. The father, in the meantime, had plenty of time to think about his prejudices and fortunately decided that his son was more important.

Early one evening seven weeks later I was called out to Auburn police station, about thirty minutes west of Sydney. When I arrived I saw a Ford F100 caged police truck parked in the driveway. The front of the truck was facing the station and the rear-caged section was facing the street, opposite a pub. Two uniform police stood at the rear of the truck next to the closed door, and Steve York, our negotiation team leader, was talking to one of these officers.

It seemed a gentleman by the name of Keith had entered the police station earlier in the evening to hand himself in. Apparently he had a number of outstanding warrants requiring him to pay a substantial amount of money that he did not have. Instead of paying the fines he wanted to go to gaol to 'cut out the warrant', that is, spend a few days in prison instead of paying the money.

The warrants were found and Keith was taken into custody; the caged truck was brought around and Keith put in the back to be taken to gaol. When the police were backing out of the drive, one of them noticed a movement in the rear. Keith was holding a knife which had been taped to his back. The officer immediately stopped the truck and with his partner went to open the rear door. Keith screamed at them that he had a knife and would stab them if they tried to pull him out, and that he also wanted to kill himself. That was when the police locked the door again and asked for specialist help from the TOU, including negotiators.

Steve and I were the only ones there. He asked me, 'Well, are you right to be the primary negotiator?' I hadn't been asked before, and was only due to undertake the second part of my training the following month, so I felt pretty anxious at the prospect. At the same time, I was honoured that Steve was confident I could do the job. Face-to-face negotiations are considered the most difficult and the most dangerous, as the negotiator is in full view of the subject. I knew I needed to be very careful of my body language and to be sure that my actions remained consistent with my words.

The Tactical team, who? had just arrived and were organising their equipment, gave me the go-ahead, so I walked over and stood about a metre away from the back of the police truck. I could just see Keith through the two small cut-outs on either side of the door, like tiny windows, and heard him muttering to himself. His face was not visible, but I had no doubt he could see mine if he chose to look.

'Hello, Keith,' I said. 'My name is Belinda and I am a police negotiator. I am here to help you.'

'Just fuck off all of you. Fuck off.'

'Keith, I can see that you are very upset ...'

'Just fuck off.'

'Keith, can you tell me why you have the knife?'

Keith yelled, 'Because I just want to die, just fuck off and leave me in peace. You're nothing but a bunch of fuckers, get fucked.'

'Keith, why do you feel this way?'

'Just fuck off, I want to die.'

'Keith, I would like to see you safely out of the truck,'

'Don't you get it? *Fuck off!*'

Not a good start, and the conversation continued like this for about an hour. I asked Keith various open questions about his life, work, family, interests, and Keith yelled obscenities. After a while I needed a break.

'Keith, I am going to speak to some other police,' I said. 'I will be back soon. I would like you to promise me you will not hurt yourself while I am gone.'

'Yeah, sure,' he replied. 'Just call out my name if you need me.'

I left the uniformed police at the rear of the truck and found Steve. Not having seen the Tactical police at the rear of the truck, I asked him where they were. He took me around the back of the police station and I could see them practising a tactical resolution – assault – using another caged truck. This was not a good scenario. Due to the confined nature of the rear of the truck, they would only be able to have one operator in at a time, so the momentum of the assault would be to Keith's advantage.

I spoke to Steve about the negotiations and asked how I was going.

'Do you want the good news or the bad news?' he said.

I gulped. 'There's bad news?'

'This is the third time he has been involved in a siege with police, and the other occasions were all tactical resolutions.' He explained that on the first occasion. Keith had gone to a service station in Ashfield, taken a petrol hose off the bowser and started spraying it around, threatening to light it. The amount of petrol flowing around and into the gutters would have caused substantial damage to the service station and the surrounding area if it had been ignited. Negotiation had failed and armed police had moved very quickly to disarm him, putting their own lives at risk. On the second occasion, Keith had been at his home unit armed with a knife and threatened suicide, and again police had been forced to risk their lives to save him.

After hearing all this, I was not feeling too confident about resolving this situation by means of the negotiation process. However, I was not yet prepared to concede. I returned to the rear of the truck, ensuring I kept my back to the pub so I wasn't distracted by the row of spectators who had gathered to watch what was happening.

'Hi Keith, I'm back, how are you going?'

We picked up right where we had left off and went on for another half hour. Eventually I had had enough of the swearing and verbal abuse.

'Keith, I have been speaking with you for some time, I have been calm and talking normally. Why are you swearing and abusing me? I am not being unkind.'

Then he said, 'My name's not Keith! It's fucking Kevin!'

I couldn't believe I had made such an elementary mistake. Nobody likes people getting their name wrong, no one. I quickly apologised to Kevin and we started to have a normal conversation about his life, his work possibilities, and family.

At one stage he wanted to go to the toilet. I immediately said, 'Kevin, if you put the knife through the window and drop it to the ground, we can open the door, let you out and take you to the toilet.' He wasn't ready to come out, believing the police would assault him, and knowing what had happened in previous sieges I could understand why. Then he said, 'Too late,' and I had to jump out of the way as the urine splashed out from underneath the rear door.

Eventually Kevin started warming to the idea of leaving the truck. As I was discovering, negotiator situations can either be resolved quickly or they can take hours. I believe the time taken depends very much on the person coming to terms with their own fears, and perhaps realising, through conversation with a negotiator, that peaceful resolution is their best or only option. If the negotiator can build up enough rapport with the person, the situation is more likely to be resolved peacefully.

It took another thirty or forty minutes to convince Kevin to drop the knife through the window. I started to talk him through the next phase, explaining what would happen, including impressing upon him that I would be there. Tactical police officers were positioned near the rear of the truck at this point.

One of the Tactical police opened the door and Kevin came out and into custody. I made sure I was standing behind the Tactical police at this stage so he could see I was still there for him. It was also possible that Kevin could have another breakdown, creating another siege. If that happened other negotiators could use my report to remind him that the police had kept their word and he was unharmed. Kevin was then taken by uniform police for psychiatric assessment; the chilling thing about this is that sometimes the person is allowed to leave the hospital even before the police have made it back to the station.

I learned two lessons from this. Always confirm a person's name, and search prisoners properly before they are put into police vehicles.

There was a chilling sequel. About twelve months later I learned that Kevin had climbed up onto a pylon of the Sydney Harbour Bridge and jumped to his death. I felt sad and frustrated that the system had let him down. If only someone had given him the help he so desperately needed, the outcome might have been very different.

CHAPTER

5

Not a great start to a marriage

At the end of April 1993 I went on a three-month European holiday with some girlfriends. This was my final fling as an unmarried woman: Rob and I had arranged our wedding for November. After a twenty-five-day Contiki trip around various places, I went to Switzerland to visit one of my best friends, who was working as an au pair. I spent some time in the Greek islands, then visited Thailand on my way home. I had a wonderful time.

In July, I returned to work at the Drug Enforcement Agency Support Unit. Once again I was asked to fill in for one of the permanent on-call negotiation teams.

On 26 August my on-call negotiator pager activated. A man had just shot and killed three people in Redfern in inner Sydney, had taken off and was now involved in a standoff with local police at Burwood about ten kilometres further west.

I had to get there fast as part of a negotiation team, and the SPG TOU was on its way.

My skin started to prickle. This was an extremely serious situation. I knew Rob was working at the Tactical Operations Unit that day and was worried that he might be coming to Burwood as well. With my mind racing and heart pumping, I put the blue light on the roof of the police car and took off for Burwood at high speed.

By the time I got to Canterbury Road, Canterbury, still travelling at high speed with lights and sirens, the on-call negotiation pager activated again. I didn't have a mobile to ring in – in those days mobile phones were quite rare, and the only ones available were very expensive and about the size of a house brick. I knew Canterbury police station was not far away; I would be able to find a phone there. When I did, I was told that the man was in custody and negotiators were being called off. I tried ringing the SPG TOU office but there was no response. I thought Rob might have been at another job, and reasoned that, if he had been involved in this situation, the offender was now in custody so all should be well. I got back in my car and started to drive back towards the city.

When I got back to the office, I did some paperwork during the afternoon and called the SPG TOU office again. Still no one was answering the phone, and there was no word from Rob. I felt that perhaps they were organising their equipment, packing it away, perhaps having a beer to debrief after the siege, a common way for police to relax after a very stressful incident.

At the end of the day I drove home to Ramsgate, where I was living with my flatmate. By now I was starting to get worried as I still hadn't had any word. I called the SPG TOU office again and finally I was able to get hold of someone. Yes, Rob and the guys were there. They were having a drink as a form of stress relief.

Rob was talking at an incredible rate, still hyped up. He had gone to Burwood and there had been a shootout with the man, who was armed. Rob was convinced he'd fired the shot that impacted and disabled the gunman's rifle. I left him to it as he needed to talk and debrief with the others. I was just relieved that he seemed fine, though even more animated than usual.

I rang the next day at work to see how he was. One of the Tactical operators answered the phone and the conversation went like this.

'Hi, it's Belinda. Is Rob there?'

'He's at the hospital.'

'Why, what's the matter?'

'He got shot, but it looks like his body armour stopped a bullet.'

I was dumbfounded. 'But I was talking to him only yesterday.'

The operator said he would find out what had happened and call me back. A short time later he came back to me: 'He's at St Vincent's Hospital, they're doing some X-rays and tests but it could have been worse. His body armour did stop the bullet.'

He said the hospital was about to release Rob, and that he should be back in the office in an hour or so. There was no need for me to rush to the hospital if he was going to be back soon.

When I got off the phone I just sat there, stunned. Rob's ballistics vest had stopped a bullet. How lucky was that? All the time I just took for granted that each time we went to a high-risk job, or any job for that matter, we would do what was required, fill out the paperwork and go home. Sure, the possibility of getting hurt or killed was all part and parcel of the work. Being confronted by such a close call, however, was a shock.

Rob had a perfectly round bruise the size of a ten-cent piece on his lower right abdomen, missing the unprotected part of his body by approximately three centimetres. He said he had indeed gone to Burwood; the man who had murdered three people was apparently about to kill a fourth. When Rob and his team arrived at the scene, local police were already involved in a shootout. The offender was shooting at police from behind a tree. It was chaotic, bullets were flying in all directions and local police had taken cover behind their vehicles. Rob and the other three Tactical police officers, seeing the danger the local police were in, quickly took up their positions and confronted the offender. Rob and the TOU operatives were armed with Heckler and Koch MP5 9mms, which they had taken because they were initially on their way to a drug buy bust, and would be working from the confined space of a vehicle. Rob would have preferred an M16 semi-automatic rifle; the offender had a high-powered 30.06 rifle and a twelve-gauge shotgun.

The Tactical operatives quickly drew fire away from the local police and towards themselves, and the man duly started firing at Rob and the other TOU police. Rob said he heard a shot and felt a heavy blow to the lower area of the right side of his stomach. However it affected him no more than that, possibly due to the adrenalin pumping through his system. Shortly after this, the suspect for some reason came out from behind the bush and towards them, still firing. They wounded him in the leg and disabled his rifle, and he surrendered and was quickly arrested.

With so much adrenalin running through his system, Rob didn't even realise he had been shot until later that night. He started suffering severe cramps and pain above his right groin and next morning he noticed the circular bruise. He went to work as usual but the cramps grew worse and he was taken to the hospital. He had suffered a severe blunt trauma wound, which had compressed his stomach and vital organs. I still cannot believe he was so lucky.

For a long time afterwards, Rob was moody and angry. For the first six months after our wedding in November 1993, we fought to the point where the marriage came close to breaking down. Rob wasn't sleeping well and he would lose his temper at the drop of a hat. I put this down to my headstrong nature and Rob's domineering one: I was one of very few people he couldn't intimidate. In retrospect, I can see now that Rob had all the symptoms of post-traumatic stress disorder. Unfortunately, we didn't realise that then, and there was no counselling provided for him.

Rob and I were extremely supportive of each other when it came to our jobs, our careers. I believe this was because we respected each other's abilities, we sought advice from each other, and we could talk to each other about our work. We felt the same concern for each other, and we both knew what went on in the world in a way that the broadcast news just doesn't convey.

The downside was that we could not get away from work; it followed us home. We were both working long, exhausting hours, Rob with the TOU and me in drug and homicide investigation: I was also working part-time as a negotiator. Either of us could be called into work at short notice, even on rest days or annual leave, and we were often called away to situations throughout the state. Recently I found out that in the mid 1990s I was the highest overtime earner in the state police force.

Most of our friends were police, except for some dear school friends of mine, and my time with them was rare and very special. Socialising with other police, however, seemed natural: we all worked hard, and we understood each other. We went to work functions, dinners, even sporting events and fixtures together. Rob introduced me to triathlons, we trained together and had a lot of fun.

Marriage, at that time, had curbed my wild drinking ways after the deaths of Tim and Dana. In fact, Rob had had a steadying influence on me: after these tragedies I had continued my cycle of late nights and drinking. Rob and I both enjoyed a social drink but our increased workloads and on-call periods at that time meant that alcohol wasn't an issue. However, work was. We did not see each other at work often, sometimes only when we were called out to high-risk operations together. When we did have time together outside work we were often tired and decided to spend a night at home. We had occasional trips away in the Hunter Valley, Blue Mountains, or Central Coast, mainly on weekends, and we always stayed in lovely, romantic accommodation. Apart from our honeymoon in Vanuatu, we never again went overseas together.

After one particular afternoon shift Rob, due home about 11.30pm, didn't arrive. He would always contact me if he was working overtime, so I started to worry. I couldn't sleep. I couldn't contact him and when I tried ringing the office there was nobody there. About 7am the next morning he turned up at the front door. He was in a foul mood and one of the legs of his jeans was ripped to shreds. Apparently his team had had an urgent last-minute call from the Crime Squad to help them carry out a high-risk search warrant at a bikies' clubhouse. There had been no time for them to change into the overalls they usually wore to such incidents, and they had left the office quickly to get into position. The operation had continued into the night, which meant that he couldn't contact me until the job had finished. While they were moving to surround the premises a police dog had latched on to Rob's right calf, ripping his jeans. He was furious: they had been a good pair. I couldn't have cared less about the jeans, I was just thankful he was all right.

CHAPTER
6

The De Gruchy murders

By mid 1994 I had spent almost five years at the DEA. It was standard policy for staff to be transferred out after a maximum of five years there, and I was ready for a move. When an opportunity arose to transfer to the Major Crime Squad South I didn't hesitate. Unfortunately the only vacancy available was in the Drug Unit. I had already had enough of drug investigation and wanted to try something new. I wanted to go to the Squad's Homicide Unit. However, the opportunity to get a 'foot in the door' at the Major Crime Squad was too good to pass up – and worth spending almost two years in drug investigation again before I was able to transfer to Homicide.

As a detective who was a Homicide investigator, I believed I had reached the pinnacle of my investigative career. I felt it was a privilege to investigate the death of one human being at the hand of another, to use all available resources at my investigative disposal, to prepare briefs of evidence for the Supreme Court in helping bring murderers to justice.

The investigation of a murder is very challenging. The first forty-eight hours are particularly demanding because there is usually an overwhelming influx of information from potential witnesses and suspects, with clues and evidence. Evaluating the information and deciding on which avenues of inquiry to follow and which tools of investigation to use is extremely interesting. The downside to homicide investigation, of course, is exposure to sickeningly violent human behaviour and some of the most horrific crimes imaginable.

The inspector in charge of Homicide was one of the most experienced homicide investigators in Australia. He had been an investigator in the case of Anita Cobby, the twenty-six-year-old nurse who had been abducted, raped and murdered in western Sydney in February 1986 – still considered one of Australia's more horrific crimes. Five men were found guilty of her murder.

At 8am I was on duty for my first shift in Homicide and busy moving some of my files from the Drug Squad over to my new desk. About 11am, the phone rang.

'Good morning, Detective Neil, Homicide Unit,' I answered for the first time. 'How can I help you?'

The voice on the other end said, 'This is John Smith from the *Daily Telegraph*. Has Homicide sent anybody down to that triple murder at Albion Park?'

Yeah right, I thought and looked around the office for the practical joker to appear. No sign of anyone playing a joke, yet none of the investigators knew anything about this case. I told the reporter I needed to make further inquiries and ended the call. It was unusual to be contacted by the press prior to police; normally local police contacted us as soon as they had been to a crime scene to assess what resources might be required. In this case, however, reporters more than likely intercepted initial police radio calls to the scene.

Local police confirmed that three people had been murdered at Albion Park Rail about an hour and a half south of Sydney. A short time later I was asked to go to Warilla police station, which covered the Albion Park area, with other Homicide police to assist local investigators. We were told that the officer in charge of the investigation would brief us when we arrived.

I had never been to a murder scene before. The only bodies I had encountered, in general duties at Waverley, had been people who died of natural causes. As probationers, we had been taken to the city morgue and shown the room where autopsies were held, but none were being conducted that day. Even when I was in drug investigation I had not seen anyone who had died from an overdose. I felt a little apprehensive. I was one of four Homicide investigators and I knew that because this was my first day in the unit I would be expected to watch what happened closely, learn, and give help where needed.

At the police station we were told that Jennifer De Gruchy, her thirteen-year-old daughter Sarah and fifteen-year-old son Adrian had been brutally murdered in their home at Albion Park Rail. Matthew De Gruchy, the eighteen-year-old brother of Sarah and Adrian, had found the bodies of his mother and sister. He was to be interviewed by the police, and so was Wayne De Gruchy, Jennifer's husband and the children's father.

After preliminary inquiries it was believed that Wayne was not involved in the murder. Questioning him so closely after what had happened might seem callous, however, while police are generally respectful in dealing with bereaved relatives, family members cannot immediately be ruled out as potential suspects. At the beginning of a murder investigation everyone is a suspect.

I was asked to take a statement from Wayne. It took nearly five hours. We talked about the family, his work, where he had been the previous evening. He said he had stayed at his parents' home in Sydney, something he often did because he worked in the city. He said he had last spoken with his wife Jennifer on the phone the previous evening. His son Matthew had wanted to use the car to visit his girlfriend; either Wayne or Jennifer – Wayne wasn't sure who – had refused permission.

The crime scene was a typical single-storey brick suburban home. From the front of the house, nothing looked out of place except for the presence of a number of police cars. We went into the main bedroom, and that was where normality ended. This was the room where Jennifer's body had been found. It was no longer there, having been taken to the morgue. The bed and a pillow were covered in blood, so much blood that I knew her facial injuries would have been horrific.

The next bedroom, obviously Sarah's, had a bloodstained pillow on the single bed. I had been told she too had suffered severe wounds to the head and arms. There was a Walkman on the floor next to her bed; I imagined her lying there listening to music, not hearing what was happening in her mother's room. Someone had put a pillow over her face and, while she raised her arms to defend herself, she had been brutally struck again and again.

Did the killer know Sarah? Had the pillow been put over her head to prevent her from seeing the killer's face? I felt sick. I couldn't imagine what kind of person could do that. However, I knew that if I wanted to do my job properly I would have to divorce myself from the horror all around me. *Look at this crime scene as a canvas*, I told myself. *Don't consider the human factor, don't allow feelings to get in the way. There are no bodies, just look for the clues to tell us what took place here.*

This was more easily said than done, especially when we went into the garage. There were human teeth on the floor, blood spatters on the ceiling. On the floor was an open jerry-can, the smell of petrol intermingling with the smell of blood. This was where the first officer on the scene had discovered the body of fifteen-year-old Adrian. Like his sister, Adrian had suffered severe head wounds and lacerations. Someone had also poured petrol over him, perhaps to try and set him alight. Had Adrian caught this person in the act of killing his mother and sister?

The rest of the crime scene provided some interesting clues. There was evidence of a burglary, but some obviously valuable items such as a jewellery box containing earrings, necklaces and rings had been left untouched. A video recorder had gone, and taken out so neatly from the television cabinet that three videos standing up on either side were not disturbed. The floors had been wiped down and pieces of carpet cut out from the main bedroom. Compared with the frenzied attacks that had taken place, this kind of care was bizarre. The whole crime scene appeared to be a poorly conceived effort by someone to make it look like a robbery gone wrong.

Even though the bodies had been removed, my mental images of what had happened to those three people were probably more horrific than if I had seen the bodies myself. I kept going over and over them, and was almost relieved when it was time to leave the house at about one in the morning.

To say this first day in the Homicide Unit had been an eye-opener for me was an understatement. The De Gruchy case supplied one of the most horrendous crime scenes I ever saw in my entire police career. Aspects of this crime would come back to haunt me years later.

The next morning at nine I went into the inspector's office with the supervisor to make my report. The boss looked at me and said, 'Well you've been blooded.' Not a great choice of words, I thought, but I took it to mean I had been initiated into the world of Homicide. He added that he heard I had done well. I hadn't realised I was being watched so closely.

My job that day was to go to Glebe morgue for the post-mortems of Jennifer, Sarah and Adrian De Gruchy. This was fine with me; I had no idea what I was in for.

When I got there I was shown into the autopsy room, where they gave me a hospital gown to put over my clothes. That day I was wearing a dark green skirt with a cream blouse and a matching dark green jacket. Amazing the things you remember, particularly those you might prefer to forget. Besides Homicide investigators, there were crime scene officers to photograph and record findings made by the forensic pathologist, Dr Alan Cala. I had dealings with Dr Cala a number of times over the next few years, and always found him very professional and intelligent. The autopsy room had rows of stainless steel benches, with taps at the ends. Three of these benches were together, with a body on each of them.

Adrian and Sarah De Gruchy were to be autopsied first. The pathologist examined their bodies, and then their heads were shaved to ascertain the exact damage to their skulls. Fifteen-year-old Adrian's white skin was covered in red slashes. There were twenty-one to his head and neck. His face and the base of his skull were grossly fractured, and there were also fractures to his cheekbone and jawbone. Dr Cala located teeth, roots and all, in Adrian's nose cavity. His torso had bruises like tram tracks. (Sarah and Jennifer had similar bruising, which indicated the type of weapon used.) The skin on his arms was peeling, consistent with petrol being poured on him to set him alight. I was appalled by the viciousness of the attack on this young boy, and could see that the others present were similarly shocked.

The ten lacerations to Sarah's beautiful young face and head were startling red slits against her pale white skin. Like Adrian, she had suffered fractures to her skull, forehead, right side and base of her skull. What made me feel especially sick were the defensive wounds to her right arm. They were in the same tram track pattern as Adrian's and it looked as if the weapon used could have been a wheel brace or tyre lever. The investigating police were told this so they could start looking for the murder weapon as a matter of urgency.

Jennifer De Gruchy was a slight, small woman with dark hair. Her face had been bashed in, all bloodied and bruised. When the pathologist examined her skull, he had difficulty working out the number of strikes as compared to the bone fractures. The wounds to her face were so severe that he believed that the weapon had been either a sledgehammer or wheel brace.

Whoever had killed this family had really gone berserk and inflicted incredible injuries. I still couldn't comprehend that a human being could do this to another human being. Being exposed to the sheer physical violence that this crime scene provided was a real shock. This was no *CSI* or any other TV crime show. These were real bodies with real blood and wounds. The De Gruchy crime scene was so awful that one police officer who attended it never returned to work.

I finished at 8.30pm. I was exhausted and went home. Thank heavens Rob was there; I needed to talk to someone about what I had seen, to try and process the horror of such violence. I was too tired to eat; all I needed was to feel clean. I hung my dark green jacket over a chair in the dining room and hung up the matching skirt, sure they had another day's wear in them before needing to be dry cleaned. The rest of my clothes I left lying on the bathroom floor while I jumped into the shower. The hot water felt wonderful, washing away the events of the day.

The next morning I woke up to get ready for work to find that a very strange unpleasant smell seemed to be all through the unit. It was my jacket, reeking of formaldehyde.

Some weeks later two bags and some loose items were found in a local dam, not far from where Matthew De Gruchy's girlfriend lived. They included the video recorder, clothing and other things taken from the De Gruchy house, as well as pieces of carpet, Jennifer De Gruchy's driver's licence and a calculator labelled with Adrian De Gruchy's name. Of most interest was a torn-up note in handwriting identified as Matthew De Gruchy's. It was headed 'Sarah, Adrian and Mum' and described a plan to remove incriminating physical evidence from the scene as well as ways of making it look as though Matthew, the other son, had been assaulted. The tyre lever from Jennifer De Gruchy's car, possibly the murder weapon, was never found.

I had seen Matthew De Gruchy at the police station: a slight, insipid, even weedy boy, not very tall with dark hair. It was hard to fathom how he could contain such aggression and cause so much damage. In June 1996 he was arrested and charged with the murders of his mother, sister and his brother. He never made any admissions about the murders or his actions. He was later convicted and sentenced to three concurrent terms of imprisonment of twenty-eight years with a minimum of twenty-one years. He is not eligible for parole until 2017.

I returned to work in the Homicide office. According to my police issue duty book, I had conversations with Wayne De Gruchy and his brother and went back to the crime scene with other police officers, but I have no recollection of this. Mentally I had shut down. However, I carried the crime scene with me, my own personal horror movie in full technicolor. The shocking images remained etched in my mind, part of a growing and gruesome mental scrapbook.

7

The case of kim meredith

On the morning of Saturday 23 March 1996, just ten days after the De Gruchy murders, I was about to enjoy a well-deserved day off when the home phone rang. It was Detective Sergeant Wayne Hayes asking me whether I was available to travel to Albury to assist local detectives in investigating the brutal murder of a young woman.

I said I was. I was no longer involved in the De Gruchy investigation and had no other pressing work commitments. This was not only another major case, it would also enable me to work with Wayne, a highly regarded investigator; if I said no I might never be asked again. I quickly packed a bag, Wayne picked me up and we drove to Albury, about six and a half hours south-west of Sydney with a stop for lunch.

We went to the police command post near the intersection of Swift and Macauley streets: easy to find because of the cars with the revolving blue lights and the blue-and-white checkered crime-scene tape. We parked and walked towards the young constable who was guarding the crime scene. He quickly stood up, looking ill at ease; we were not in uniform so he probably thought we were journalists. When we showed our police ID and explained who we were, he produced the crime-scene register and we signed in.

The police had floodlit the scene of the crime, which was not large, just a small car park and yard at the rear of an office block. A door to the rear of the office block had a light above it and next to that was a grassed area, a lattice screen and bushes near a fence.

One of the first things I saw was a large pool of blood in the car park with a trail leading from it in the shape of a figure eight. The body of nineteen-year-old Kim Meredith had been dragged behind the lattice screen then back to the door, where she was found. She was almost naked, wearing only a pair of socks. Shoe prints were found in her blood. Her clothes had apparently been pulled off behind the lattice screen, with her bra, panties and shoes dumped behind it. Her blouse had been thrown up on the roof of the office block. The jacket and jeans she had been wearing were found in a disused toilet to the rear of the adjoining premises, and her handbag was in the same area.

I kept looking towards the large pool of blood while I tried to understand what had happened. I knew that she had had her throat slashed, and if the wound was as severe as I had been told, severing major arteries, there should have been a blood spray pattern, but there wasn't. The only explanation appeared to be that she had been held face down like an animal while her throat was cut so that the blood would simply pour out straight down on the ground rather than arcing up in the air. It was a horrible image.

After we had finished examining the crime scene, we went to the morgue at the Albury Base Hospital to view Kim's body. There we met Detective Mark Smith, the officer in charge of the investigation. After seeing what had been done to the De Gruchy family, I thought I would have been better prepared for what followed. I now don't believe anything can really prepare you to see the damage one human being can inflict on another.

Kim Meredith was lying on her back on a metal hospital trolley when I saw her. The first thing I noticed was her waxen pale smooth skin and then I saw that her head had been almost severed from her body and the skin around the wound curled at a weird angle. There were twigs and leaf litter in her hair, and blood and abrasions all over her body from where she had been dragged around after her death. There was also what looked like a bite mark on one of her nipples. Her killer had wiped faeces over her stomach, a very distinctive colour against her pale skin.

It's just a body and the spirit has left the body; it's just a body and the spirit has left the body, I said to myself over and over as I stared at her wounds and made myself breathe. I had to try to forget that the body lying on the trolley was a human being so I could concentrate on investigating her death.

After viewing Kim Meredith's body we went to Albury police station and spoke with other investigators. We discovered that Kim had been studying business management and hospitality part-time at La Trobe University and that she had a casual job as a bar assistant at the Commercial Hotel. On the previous evening she had worked a shift at the hotel from

8.30pm till sometime after midnight. When she finished she drove her car to another hotel, the Terminus, to meet friends. At some stage she left the Terminus Hotel – she must have gone on foot because her car was still parked near the hotel – and it is believed she was heading towards Sodens Hotel to meet up with other friends. She never made it.

The detectives from Albury had been involved in the investigation since the early hours of the morning after a local security guard found her body. Our role was not to take over the murder investigation but to provide investigative expertise, to assist in the investigation and aid local detectives. We spent much of our time evaluating various pieces of information that were flowing in to the police. We finished at 1.30am.

About nine the next morning Wayne and I had a briefing with other police to discuss the information we had, look at investigative strategies, and see where the investigation was headed. The Albury detectives were in charge of the primary victim care, that is, they were liaising with Kim Meredith's family, her mother, father and brother, and keeping them up to date with the progress of the investigation.

One of the investigators told me that Kim's mother had wanted to know how long Kim's body had been at the crime scene. It seemed an odd question, and its significance did not strike me until years later – here was a mother wanting to know how long her child had lain naked and alone, an anguished mother unable to comfort her child, even in death.

During the day information continued to flow in from a number of sources, particularly concerning a local man named Graham Mailes. He was well known to Albury police, having a lengthy criminal history involving assault and carrying a knife. Mailes had been seen in Albury in the early hours of the evening on the night of the murder, but was now on his way back to Forbes, 370 kilometres north of Albury, where he lived with his aunt and her family.

A man said that in the early hours of the morning after the murder Mailes had asked his help in getting money from an ATM. When we checked with the bank we found that Kim Meredith's credit card had been used twice, at 2.40 and 2.41am, in an attempt to get the same sums of money that the witness said Mailes had tried to obtain. This happened twenty minutes before her body was discovered. Another witness saw Mailes in an agitated state at a men's shelter and had noticed what appeared to be blood on his jeans. We also talked to one of Mailes's friends. It became imperative to talk to Mailes himself.

About 9.30 that night four of us drove at high speed to Forbes to find Graham Mailes, arriving at about one in the morning. We had little time to rest; at 6am we presented ourselves at Forbes police station, where the local detectives would, we hoped, lead us to our prime suspect. The house was on the outskirts of town and Kate, Mailes's aunt, answered the door, followed by Mailes himself.

Graham Mailes was a sinister individual, not a man anyone would like to see in a dark alley. Taller than me with a slim but muscular build, he had ginger blonde short hair and a severe cleft palate.

Kate took Wayne and me into the laundry and showed us a pile of Mailes's clothes thrown on the floor. She later surrendered a pair of his blue Stubbies jeans – and a blue collared shirt, later identified as Kim Meredith's. Both garments were heavily stained with blood. Mailes agreed to come back to Forbes police station to be interviewed. During the interview he told us he had spent the night of the murder with his girlfriend Debra and had left for Forbes the following morning.

We took Mailes to the local medical centre so a doctor could take blood samples from him, as well as hair from his head and fingernail scrapings. I recall him wincing when a couple of hairs were pulled out and I couldn't help thinking about the pain inflicted upon Kim Meredith. Wayne provided Mailes with another pair of shoes and the joggers and socks Mailes was wearing were taken as evidence. Kim Meredith's blood was later identified on the joggers and the shoe impressions at the crime scene were also found to match the joggers Mailes had been wearing.

Unfortunately, all this DNA testing took several days and Mailes had been allowed to leave the police station. After he left, we continued painstakingly working through evidence, including his purchase of a lock knife on the night of the murder and a Guess watch he had in his possession.

The next morning, Tuesday 26 March Wayne and I, together with the two investigators from Albury, drove out to the home at Forbes where Mailes lived. He was mustering sheep in a paddock. After Wayne had offered to help him he consented to come back to the police station provided he was given a lift home, which was agreed. Wayne and Detective Smith started helping Mailes move the sheep and I chose to drive behind them. I was wearing cream-coloured high-heeled shoes, definitely not the best choice of footwear for walking through a dusty paddock with a suspected murderer.

We still didn't have enough evidence to charge him with murder and we desperately needed results from the blood examinations. We needed to take a number of exhibits, including the lock knife and the Guess watch now identified as Kim Meredith's, for examination at the government's Department of Analytical Laboratories at Lidcombe approximately 350 kilometres away. We drove there next morning, delivered the exhibits and drove back towards Albury: a long day of driving, about 700 kilometres.

The next day we did a 'video run-around' with police from the Video Unit who had travelled to Albury. A bus had been organised to convey investigators, Video Unit officers, and Mailes and his aunt. She had been invited as support for Mailes, as we believed that while he seemed very street smart, he had a mild intellectual disability. The video run-around meant visiting various places around Albury, including where Mailes's girlfriend lived, and making recordings. This took the better part of the day and by the time we had reached the car park, the scene of the murder, the media, including television cameras, were well and truly present. The media can be a great ally. They can be a very useful tool, for example in enlisting public help to aid investigations. However, in certain circumstances they can be an encumbrance. In this instance, we would have preferred not to have media present to avoid spooking Mailes.

Police interviewed Mailes again and I watched from another room. When testimony from witnesses appeared to contradict what he had said, including his girlfriend Debra's declaration that she had not seen him for more than a year and had never lived at the residence Mailes pointed out, he simply said they were wrong or lying.

Before long the interview room door opened and Mark, who had been questioning Mailes, came out, leaving the door open. It was only a small room, about 2 x 2.5 metres square, with Mailes sitting sitting directly in front of the small table on which was the electronic recording device including video and tape recorder, with two chairs opposite. Wayne was sitting on one of these; the other was empty as Mark had left the room.

Mailes appeared agitated, very unsettled; his head was shaking, his face was red. Mark came over and explained to his aunt Kate that he had just told Mailes he was about to charge him with murder, and asked her to come into the room to see whether her presence might calm him. She went in with him.

All of a sudden Mailes pulled his right arm back, clenched his fist and drove it straight towards the left side of Mark's face. Next minute the two of them were on the floor struggling. Kate ran out of the room while Wayne rushed in to help Mark. They were quickly joined by other police who had been watching on closed-circuit TV in another room. Eventually Mailes was restrained, though it took a number of police to overpower him, and he was handcuffed and led away. He had a bleeding cut above his right eye and I was amazed when he complained about the pain: again, it was hard not to consider the fear and agony Kim Meredith must have suffered.

When I returned to Sydney the following day I was drained. Two days later I was providing Homicide assistance to local investigators at Sutherland regarding a suspected paedophile murder and I really needed some days off. I was rostered for five rest days, which I was looking forward to, just spending some time with Rob and not doing very much.

On my last rest day I had a phone call from Detective Senior Constable Robert Allison at the Homicide Unit. Mailes, who was currently at Long Bay prison hospital, wanted to speak with police about the Kim Meredith murder. Mark in Albury would normally have handled this, but he wouldn't be able to get to Sydney for six or seven hours and felt the matter was urgent. Could Wayne and I do the interview? Wayne was on holiday in Queensland, so it was down to me. I really wanted to do this right; it was my first Homicide interview and I did not want to do it by myself. Fortunately Detective Robert Allison, who was more experienced, was available.

I headed into the Homicide office trying to collect my thoughts and wrap them back around the Kim Meredith murder investigation. I found a portable Electronic Recorded Interview with Suspected Person (ERISP) machine and away we went.

Long Bay Correctional Centre is based at Malabar in Sydney, and its hospital is a maximum-security facility. After passing through numerous security checks, we were shown to a room where I could set up the ERISP machine. A short time later, Mailes was brought in.

After introducing ourselves to Mailes, and confirming that he wanted to talk about the murder of Kim Meredith, I launched into procedural questions and confirmed that he understood what was about to happen, including that he would be given a complete copy of the interview on audio cassette. Then I asked the question we all wanted answered. 'Can you tell me why you wish to speak to us?'

He replied, 'Why? I didn't done the murder. I know who done it.' He added, 'But when the murder happened I was there.'

Over the next two and a half hours Mailes dealt in excruciating detail with every bit of evidence against him in the police fact sheet tendered to court. In his initial police interview he had denied a witness's statement that he had been with another friend, Damien, about midnight and they had bought hot dogs. Now he said they had been together. After midnight, he said he and his best mate, Tony, went for drinks at the Terminus Hotel, the last place that Kim Meredith was seen alive. (Though they were allegedly best friends, Mailes had said that prior to that night he had not seen Tony for four years.) About 2.30am Tony had suddenly left the hotel and Mailes followed him. He saw a girl walking up a laneway – it was one that the police had shown Mailes during the video run-around – and Tony attacked her.

Mailes said, 'He had his hands around her throat, I was a hundred yards away and I said, "What're you doing?" He took her across the road, he took the knife out, that's when I saw the knife in his hand, that's when he slashed her, went *swwwwwt* real quick. I seen blood bursting out, right, and that's when I walked off.' Mailes explained the blood on his own jeans and shirt by saying that, because Tony had been wearing shorts and was therefore barred from the pub, he had given him his own jeans and short-sleeved shirt and put on some black tracksuit pants he found in a Vinnies bin. Tony was about his own height but slimmer.

Various other statements changed throughout the interview. At one point Mailes said he saw Tony dragging the girl across the road and he himself stood opposite acting as a lookout for Tony in case somebody came. He remained adamant that as soon as he saw Tony cut the girl's throat he had left the crime scene and Tony caught up with him five minutes later. This, of course, did not fit with the length of time taken to drag Kim Meredith's body around the crime scene, undress her, hide her belongings in various areas then leave her body, naked except for socks, lying underneath the light.

He said Tony had given him Kim Meredith's Guess watch, but also threatened him if he told anyone what had happened. He then asked for his own clothes back and put them on, even though they were covered in blood, and went home.

Mailes agreed that he had sometimes lied in his previous interviews. However, he still denied having Kim Meredith's credit card and using it at the ATM in the early hours of the morning, even though he had been identified. About the footprints found near the body, he said they must have been Tony's as he himself had never gone near the body, however, he couldn't escape the fact that his own shoes had been stained with Kim Meredith's blood.

At the conclusion of the interview my head was pounding with a full-blown migraine. When I read the transcript later, I saw that I had asked Mailes at least eleven times how his mate had been holding Kim when he cut her throat. Usually you ask an important question two or three times throughout the interview if not satisfied with the answer; to ask as many times as I did is not particularly professional, but it does indicate my state of mind.

The next day, 10 April, I was back at work and continuing inquiries. We were contemplating wiring up a family member whom Mailes had asked to see, and who had agreed to be part of the investigation. I rang the Office of the Solicitor at police headquarters and asked a solicitor whom I knew from my Drug Squad days to arrange the affidavit necessary to use a listening device.

When the affidavit had been granted, we wired up Mailes's relative and Wayne and I took her to Long Bay. Wayne and I waited in another room while the meeting took place. When it was over, we took Mailes's relative to our office to get her statement. Mailes had apparently repeated what he told me: Tony had committed the murder.

The next day Wayne and I travelled back to Albury and continued our investigations. Among other things, we went to every clothing bin in Albury to see if Mailes's story checked out in any way, especially as he had said he climbed into the clothing bin to get black track pants. We found that only certain bins could be accessed in the way he had described.

Mailes had been staying at Quamby House on the night of the murder, and we spoke to the other residents. We were trying to find Tony. Taxi records and a carer's evidence showed he had spent the weekend with his girlfriend Gillian. Both Tony and Gillian had intellectual disabilities. Tony was exonerated.

In early June we needed to return to Forbes and Albury to carry out further investigations. Wayne and I had intended to go together, as we would achieve more in the least possible time. Unfortunately, budgetary constraints meant I had to go alone, and keep it short. This didn't make much sense to me, but it was pointless to argue, the work needed to be done, and so after spending most of a day at the office I drove the 370 kilometres to Forbes. I was so exhausted that I narrowly avoided a collision after running off the road. After a day's work in Forbes I drove on to Albury, another 380 kilometres.

Later that year Mark Smith in Albury notified me that the committal hearing for Graham Mailes would be held at the Albury local court during December, nine months after the murder. This was to determine whether there was enough evidence for the matter to proceed to trial at the Supreme Court.

I drove to Albury. The following day I waited outside the courthouse but did not get into the witness box. I met Kim Meredith's parents June and Bob, who sat in the courtroom every day. They were lovely down-to-earth decent people and I thought how difficult it must have been for them to listen to the evidence, to hear how their daughter's body had been found and what her last few moments must have been like, let alone having to look at the man who had allegedly killed her.

On Friday 6 December it was my turn to give evidence. I was asked to describe the state of Kim Meredith's body and the crime scene, and also taken through my interview with Mailes. He was later committed to stand trial for the murder.

It would not be the last time I had to evoke these awful memories. Almost three years after the murder I gave evidence at the Supreme Court in Sydney for Mailes's fitness hearing. This, which takes place before a judge, is to determine whether or not an accused person is mentally fit to stand trial, whether he or she can understand the legal proceedings and the evidence and give appropriate instructions to his legal team. Mailes was found fit to stand trial for the murder of Kim Meredith; the trial would be held later in the year at Wagga Wagga.

Because of budget restrictions, I was only allowed one trip to Wagga to assist Detective Sergeant Mark Smith with pre-trial preparations. Mark did a remarkable job of organising the numerous witnesses. In May 1999 I had to give evidence and knew Kim Meredith's family – her parents and her brother - would be sitting in the gallery and would have to listen to the tape of my interview with Graham Mailes. As I sat in the witness box listening to my own questions about the way Kim had had her throat and neck cut and Mailes's replies, I could not bring myself to look towards her family. I simply could not handle seeing the pain in their faces. At the end of the day I met Bob and June for a drink at the local pub and apologised to them because they had to listen to the taped interview.

After a lengthy trial, the jury found Graham Mailes guilty of the murder of Kim Meredith. A few months later, in September, I met Mark Smith and June and Bob Meredith in Sydney for the sentencing. Judge Newman handed down a sentence of twenty-five years in prison with a minimum parole period of eighteen years. While it was not the maximum sentence we wanted – a life sentence without parole would have been preferable – it afforded some closure for Kim Meredith's family. Or that's what we hoped.

CHAPTER

8

Work, sleep, callouts, work

Being a Homicide investigator meant working closely with families who had lost their loved ones under terrible circumstances. The pain these people suffer is indescribable. While I was attached to the Homicide Unit I attended at least three meetings of the Homicide Victims Support Group, founded by the parents of Anita Cobby and schoolgirl Ebony Simpson. The group offers twenty-four-hour support to families whose loved ones have been murdered. During meetings each person tells a heartbreaking story. My role was to answer any questions group members might have about police investigations.

I found these meetings incredibly sad and confronting. I listened while Anita Cobby's parents described their anguish at the loss of their beloved daughter, sexually assaulted and killed by five men. I listened to Ebony Simpson's parents

explain how their nine-year-old daughter had been kidnapped, sexually assaulted, and, bound but still alive, thrown
into a lake, where she drowned. One man had lost his six-
year-old son in tragic circumstances, then a year later his
partner had been murdered. These meetings always affected
me and I was often close to tears. How these families managed to soldier on amazed me.

In addition to Homicide investigation, I really enjoyed
working as a negotiator. Trying to change someone's mind
about committing suicide or causing harm to themselves or
someone else I found very rewarding. This was particularly
so as I was surrounded by so much death while working in
Homicide; the opportunity to save a life was incredibly satisfying. It made my workload a lot more demanding in comparison with other investigators, but I never considered giving
up my role as a negotiator. It never occurred to me that the
type of work I was involved in, together with my workload,
would have a major impact on my mental health.

Whilst I was still involved with the Kim Meredith murder, I
worked on other cases. On 1 April 1996, having just returned
home from Albury after the initial Meredith investigation, I
started work with Task Force Honegger, based at Sutherland
police station, investigating the murder of a suspected paedophile at Woronora south of Sydney.

One of the first things I did was go out to the crime scene,
a house tucked away along a bush track. The body appeared
to have been there for a month or more. It had not been a
pretty sight for the initial investigating police; thankfully it
had been taken to the morgue before I got there. The first
thing I noticed when I entered the house was the stench. It is
difficult to describe the smell of a body that has been lying
dead for a month, even if it has been removed; the waft that

hit me was like rotting meat mingled with the sickeningly sweet smell of blood. There was a massive bloodstain on the floor where the body had lain. The smell was overwhelming and inescapable and I was grateful to finally leave that house. I spent the next two days at Sutherland. Initial inquiries indicated the potential suspect and possible victim of paedophilia had left the country.

Over the next fortnight I continued with inquiries on the Meredith murder, arrested a man from one of my old drug investigations, travelled to Goulburn Police Academy to assist as a role-player on a negotiators' course being held there and took nearly a week of rest days, not necessarily in that order. On Friday 3 May, I went out on the town, specifically to Oxford Street, Darlinghurst, on a girls' night out, and enjoyed way too many drinks. I really needed to let off some steam after the last few hectic weeks.

The following Wednesday I learned from my Homicide supervisor Dave that a young woman had disappeared from Oxford Street a few days earlier and concern for her safety was mounting. I went to the Sydney Police Centre, where I was briefed.

On Friday 3 May Paula Brown, a thirty-year-old Sydney hairdresser, described by her friends as happy, bubbly, friendly and full of life, had dinner with some workmates then continued on drinking at the Burdekin Hotel, Oxford Street, Darlinghurst. She then disappeared. There were varying reports of last sightings. Her boss had last seen her alive about midnight, witnesses said they had seen her get into a taxi in Oxford Street about 2.30am but shortly afterwards noticed her walking back past the front of the Burdekin. Staff in Hungry Jack's restaurant on Oxford Street said they had seen her about 3.45am.

My skin crawled. I had been on a girls' night out the very same evening. Paula and I had both drunk too much and walked along Oxford Street. At least I had made it home safe.

I spent most of the next day going to various shops to buy copies of the clothes Paula had worn on the evening of 3 May according to her friends. The zebra print miniskirt and black lace shirt came from Portman's, the black platform shoes from Scooters. We took statements from her friends and set up a mannequin wearing Paula's clothes in Oxford Street, hoping to jog the memories of potential witnesses. We also set up a mobile police unit in Oxford Street.

That night I finished late, but soon after I was called out to a negotiator job. I have no idea now what this job entailed, only that my duty book indicated I finished duty at 2.30am. I was so overwhelmed by work at that stage that I didn't record where I had gone, only when.

On Sunday 12 May 1996, nine days after she disappeared, the body of Paula Brown was found in a small area of bushland near a car park in Penrhyn Road Botany. Sometime after 5pm Dave picked me up from home and we drove to the crime scene. Other Homicide investigators and crime scene officers were already there. Because it was already dark, lights had been set up.

The crime scene was sickening. Paula's body was on all fours. Her zebra print miniskirt had been pushed up and her underpants or pantyhose were down around her knees, indicating that she might have been sexually assaulted. She had severe head injuries from multiple blows to her head. I saw a liquid substance on her leg which we later found out was the work of ants. She had obviously been left in the scrubland for some days, most likely soon after she disappeared.

I felt cold and shocked that anyone could have left her like this. They could have pulled down her skirt or covered her in a blanket to give her some dignity in death. She appeared to have been thrown out of a car and just dumped. I could not believe that someone would have such little regard for a human life.

A few days later I bumped one of my old Drug Squad supervisors who used to work in the Homicide Unit, and told him about the number of homicides I had been involved in over the past couple of months. He told me that when he had been at the Unit he had had to deal with one homicide in eighteen months. I couldn't believe it; I had been to four homicides in two months.

About 12.30am on the evening the body of Paula Brown was discovered, my negotiator on-call pager activated. I'd forgotten I was still on call and as I was still at Mascot police station and there was nothing further I could do, I was free to attend the callout. The Duty Operations Inspector (DOI) told me there was a siege situation in Ward Avenue, Potts Point.

I was still hyped from the crime scene and now I had another surge of adrenalin as I sped to Potts Point. The subject was believed to be armed and had barricaded himself in an upstairs home unit. No contact had been made with him. Over the next five hours we used all manner of devices to try and start a dialogue, including a karaoke machine and megaphone, but all we managed to do was wake up the neighbours and bore the Tactical police. Because we believed the suspect had a firearm, a remote-controlled bomb disposal robot was sent in to establish if he was still in the unit. This robot was equipped with a mechanical arm, CCTV, bolt cutters, and could even carry a shotgun. At 6.35am it was confirmed that nobody was home. In this case it appeared that someone made the initial triple 000 emergency call, however, the suspect had left prior to the arrival of police.

For safety reasons it was always necessary to follow the protocols to establish whether someone was home before Tactical police entered. Once the unit had been cleared I went back to Kings Cross police station for a quick operational debriefing, then home to bed. I did not go into work that day as I had only finished at 7am.

Later in May, I was having a discussion with my supervisor about needing time to complete a number of drug briefs of evidence for upcoming trials. Suddenly I burst into tears. I didn't feel upset, and we hadn't been talking about anything sad or distressing, but my crying was out of control. I excused myself and ran to the bathroom. What was wrong with me? This had never happened before and I was mortified.

I finally stopped crying, cleaned myself up and returned to the Homicide office. Thankfully few investigators were there and no one made a comment about my actions. I returned to my desk and continued working on the briefs of evidence I had to finish.

From 19 to 26 June I had another week on call as a negotiator. These extracts from my police duty book show my workload during this time.

Saturday 22.6.96
Rest Day 2
On Duty   1.30am
Off Duty   5am
3 hours overtime submitted to SPG
Called out as Negotiator to Sydenham Road, Marrickville re John Smith DOB 01.01.67 firing shots. Arrest made by TOU.

Tuesday 25.6.96
On Duty 4am
Off Duty 5pm
4 hours overtime submitted to SPG
On duty 4am Liverpool Police Station see Detective
Goodwin, travel to Bowral, see Senior Sergeant Steinborn
and Constable Peters, briefing. Then to Bundanoon police
station attend to duties re negotiators, then to vicinity
P**** Road, Bundanoon, attend to duties as primary
negotiator. Then job complete. Return to Bundanoon
Police re equipment. Then to Bowral re debrief. Meal
10.30am–11am. Return to Sydney and continue duties in
Homicide office regarding listening device operation re
Graham Mailes, and drug trial.

Wednesday 26.6.96
On Duty 3.15am
As negotiator called out to H***** Place, Dural re Mark
Smith. Called off. Attend location see other negotiators.
Off Duty 5.15am
On Duty 8am
Off Duty 5pm
On Duty 8am
Homicide Unit, Major Crime Squad South

These early morning callouts were the most difficult. The
instant the pager was activated, the adrenalin kicked in so
by the time I contacted the DOI to find out the details of the
job and I was in the car ready to go, all my senses were alert
and my brain was already thinking about what needed to be
done on arrival. If the job was called off en route it was very
difficult to calm down and go back to sleep.

About 8pm on 4 August the on-call pager activated. A man was going berserk with a knife in a ground-floor unit at Fairfield. I arrived with lights and sirens to find that the Tactical police were setting up. Mark Goodwin, known as Goody, was the negotiation team leader, I was the primary negotiator. Once the Tactical police were in position I was ready to make the first phone call. I rang the number and the man answered, hurling abuse at me. Most of my conversations with him involved me trying to talk calmly while he screamed abuse.

Eventually he smashed the phone down, breaking it, so I needed to go face-to-face. This involved being close enough to talk to him so he could see me. I donned a ballistic vest and continued talking to him. Again it was a fairly one-sided conversation, with me still talking calmly and him swearing abuse. He was obviously destroying his property; we could hear crashing, smashing and banging inside the unit. Some of the Tactical police appeared embarrassed by the things he was screaming at me, where as I was too busy trying to think of something to say that might calm him down. In the end our strategy, after advice from a psychiatrist, was to keep him awake as long as possible. He would eventually reach a point of exhaustion and flake out.

This was one of the most gruelling negotiations I have ever undertaken. After ten hours of abuse another negotiation team came to relieve us. I saw that one of my friends, Nic, was going to have the pleasure of speaking with the man; I think she took one look at my face and realised it was not going to be easy. Nic later told me that while he was throwing furniture out of the window, he managed to grab three vintage wall ducks from their hangings and in quick succession hurled them out of the window. Flying ducks were among the last things the negotiators and the Tactical police had expected to see. The man eventually did fall asleep and was arrested.

The next afternoon, 6 August, there was another negotiator callout, this time a suicide intervention at Chatswood where a young man wanted to throw himself off a building. Fortunately, after a few hours he agreed to surrender to police and get help to set his life back on track. I was finished by 8pm.

From the moment I started at the Homicide Unit my life became a blur: work, sleep, callouts, work. I did not see much of my husband during this time as I was either away or working ridiculous hours, and I wondered whether anyone outside the police force would have accepted these working conditions.

In the middle of August I finally had some down time; I took on the job as relieving staff officer of the Major Crime Squad and undertook a Homicide course. It meant no negotiations and no late-night callouts to negotiations or homicides. Two weeks of peace, but that didn't last long.

9

Overload

On the morning of Saturday 7 September, a day off, I received a phone call at home. A short time later I was heading to Bondi to provide specialist Homicide assistance to local detectives. A British tourist had been bashed to death.

Brian Hagland, a twenty-eight-year-old backpacker, had been walking home with his girlfriend Connie Casey when two young men approached them near Campbell Parade. Twenty-two-year-old Aaron Martin had been drinking at the North Bondi RSL Club, becoming increasingly violent and aggressive. After he broke a glass pane in the toilet door and threatened to throw a stool at the bar Sean Cushman, his twenty-three-year-old mate, knew he needed to get Martin out of there. When they left the club Martin broke the glass panel of a restaurant door and smeared blood from a cut on his hand all over some walls. He was extremely abusive towards people he encountered; he was looking for a fight.

Soon the two men came across Brian and Connie, walking from the other direction. After a verbal confrontation Martin and Brian became embroiled in a serious physical fight. At one point they fell onto the roadway and Martin was strangling Brian to the point where the whites of Brian's eyes were showing. Connie, petite and fighting to save the man she loved from a drunken violent assailant, tried to get Martin off Brian by hitting him with her handbag before running to get help. Martin continued assaulting Brian and then threw or pushed him in front of a bus, and he and Cushman ran off. Brian Hagland later died of massive internal injuries.

When I arrived at Bondi police station with my work partner Wayne we were given a short briefing then a tour of the crime scene. At that stage nobody had been identified as the assailant. I met Connie, Brian's girlfriend. She was a wreck, in shock, having just watched her boyfriend of seven years being brutally beaten and strangled. Her life had been changed forever and she had no family support in Australia. The Homicide Victims Support Group was called to give her some assistance.

The fact that Brian Hagland's family were all based in England made it especially difficult for them to come to terms with what had happened. I was nominated as the Victim Liaison officer, my job being to phone Brian's family in England daily to update them on the progress of the investigation. I mainly spoke with Jane, Brian's sister, who had been delegated as the spokesperson for the family, and we had many long conversations. My job was sometimes made more difficult because the international media would sensationalise various aspects of the investigation or contact the Hagland family with information before I could tell them personally. This upset the family even further, and it was exhausting for me but I knew it was a very difficult time for them.

Over the next few days, especially after the press conference involving Connie Casey, information came pouring in from the general public eager to provide help. In one of these many calls the names of Aaron Martin and Sean Cushman came up. Both were known to police and had extensive criminal histories for dishonesty and motor vehicle offences. Martin had been convicted of a similar attack on a young man a few years earlier, when he had grabbed the young man's headphones from his head, punched him in the face so hard his nose bled; when the victim fell to the ground he kicked him in the head several times.

Within three days I was working on a listening device application for Sean Cushman's home. I rang the Office of the Solicitor at police headquarters, and knowing the pressure we were under due to the international media frenzy they provided wonderful and speedy help. Within five days the application had been approved and we installed the bug.

I had been working many fifteen-hour days and had just started an on-call week as a negotiator. Not being the officer in charge of the murder investigation, I had decided to continue with this on-call week. Within half an hour of finishing work at Bondi my negotiator pager activated; drug dealers had kidnapped an eighteen-year-old youth. I no longer felt tired, the adrenalin kicked in and my mind was going a hundred miles an hour. I headed straight to Macquarie Fields about an hour away to the southwest to meet with my team leader Goody.

We were told that the youth, Andy, had been kidnapped by some drug dealers to whom he owed money. They had telephoned Andy's father Jim and demanded $4000 for the safe return of his son, telling Jim that if he wanted Andy to return safely, he should not involve the police.

My role as the primary negotiator was to provide strategy, advice and support to Jim, since the kidnappers were not aware of police involvement. I became very focused on Jim. He was extremely upset, as what parent wouldn't be. He told me about the phone calls he had received from the kidnappers, said that Andy had been allowed to speak with him and how upset Andy had been. He broke down as he told me he had heard Andy being bashed by the kidnappers and how he could do nothing but listen to his son's screams.

We had to instill Jim with confidence that we would do everything we could to get his son back, and to give him support to speak with the kidnappers. Goody and I stayed with him until 2.30am, when another negotiation team relieved us. I felt I was abandoning Jim, but this was a high-risk situation, not a day in the office. Fatigue could severely hamper my ability to provide the right assistance to Jim and the investigation, which could result in loss of life. Even though I had been working for almost nineteen hours straight, the adrenalin pumping through my system prevented my being able to relax and fall asleep.

The next morning, after a few hours' sleep, I was back at Bondi at 8am working on the Hagland murder. I remember playing cat and mouse with the media, who were trying to follow us to obtain the latest information. I was trying to get to the listening post in a block of units near the Cushman home without being followed while not letting the media know we had methods of covert surveillance already in place.

My rest day the next day was cancelled; the kidnapping case was still in full swing. Goody and I were to go into Andy's family home at Hinchinbrook, otherwise called the 'strong-hold'. Two heavily armed Tactical police were sent in with us in case the kidnappers came to the house looking for the ransom money. I was told that Jim, his wife and another child would be home so on the way we stopped off so I could pick up some food supplies for lunch. This might sound unusual but I knew we would be entering a very stressed household and I had to ensure that Jim had eaten, as he needed his strength for the ongoing negotiations. I also wanted to try and establish some type of normality in the household, again to break the tension.

We were dropped off at the rear of their home and had to scale a 1.8-metre paling fence surrounding the sides and rear. The Tactical guys almost broke the fence because of the amount of equipment they carried. This, I am sure, could have started a small neighbourhood war. Fortunately, I only had a small gun, a handbag and food.

The family were in a very agitated state, wandering around aimlessly not knowing what to do, just waiting on the next phone call, whatever and whenever that might be. They couldn't remember when they had last eaten. Goody corralled Jim while I made lunch for the rest of the family and spoke with Jim's wife and child. We all ate lunch together, Goody and I being the surrogate family for the day. Our presence served to calm the family and allow them to regain some confidence, knowing they had help. We needed Jim to be as clear as possible in his thinking, we needed him in the best frame of mind to continue negotiating with the kidnappers.

Not long after we had eaten, Jim received a phone call from Andy saying he had been dropped off at a local petrol station and wanted his dad to come and pick him up. Andy was very distressed on the phone.

We had a very quick briefing. We were not sure if this was a setup, whether the kidnappers were with Andy or watching him and waiting to ambush Jim. It was decided that Jim would go in his car and I would sit in the front passenger seat, pretending to be an aunt who had provided the money for Andy's safe return. I would be armed with my trusty five-shot revolver. Goody and one of the tactical police officers would be hidden in the rear passenger area of the car in case things did became difficult. God only knows how they managed; it was a tight squeeze in the back and they were not small men.

I went over the plan with Jim as we drove towards the petrol station. It was a nerve-racking drive and I needed Jim to be feeling calm and confident. My hand was on my revolver, ready in case I needed to use it, and I had the bag with the money in it. We had no idea what we would find.

A short time later we arrived at the petrol station. Andy was there by himself. I scanned the area but didn't see anyone who appeared to be taking an interest in him, so Goody pulled him into the rear seat of the car on top of the guys. We drove off quickly in case the kidnappers were still around.

As soon as we were out of sight of the petrol station and it appeared we were not being followed, Goody and our Tactical officer were able to sit up properly. Introductions were made all around. Andy was a mess. When we got back to the house, he showed us where he had been bashed. His kidnappers had beaten him literally black and blue; his skinny, pale white body was covered in multicoloured bruises.

Later that evening, investigators traced the kidnappers and their organisers to a townhouse in Moorebank. Goody and I were still in the area in case negotiators were required for any high-risk arrest. Once the location of the kidnappers had been verified, we were to wait until Tactical police were in position and then, as primary negotiator, I would telephone the kidnappers.

My role now changed from one of providing strategies, advice and support to Jim in his negotiation with the kidnappers to ensuring the safe exit of each of the kidnappers out of the townhouse into police custody. With Goody standing next to me so he could relay my conversation to the Tactical police, I rang the telephone number the kidnappers had been using to contact Jim.

A male voice answered, 'Hello.'

'Hello. My name is Belinda Neil and I am a police negotiator.'

'Yes, ahh, police?'

'Yes, police. Police are investigating a kidnapping. Do you understand that?'

'Okay.'

'Police currently surround your townhouse. Do you understand that?'

The man replied, 'Yes.'

I said, 'What is your name?'

At the same time I could hear Goody's police radio advising that the front door of the townhouse had opened and an Asian man was looking out. We knew the kidnappers were armed, so to ensure that nobody was hurt as they left the townhouse they had to follow strict procedure. A wrong move could have somebody seriously injured or even killed.

In a very clear and firm voice I said, 'Do not go outside but leave the front door open. Do you understand that?'

'Yes.'

The police radio crackled again to say the front door had been left open but the Asian man had gone back inside the house, having seen the Tactical police.

I said, 'I will get you to leave the house soon but there are some things we need to discuss to ensure your safety. Do you understand that?'

He did. I again asked him his name, which he provided.

I said, 'How many people are in the house?'

He said, 'Three.'

I said, 'Can you tell me their names?'

He supplied them. I said, 'Are there any weapons in the house?'

'No, no.'

I said, 'I will get each of you to leave the house one at a time. You will be first and I will also speak to each of the others before they leave the house. Do you understand that?'

'Yes.'

I could hear other voices in the background. The man I was speaking to said something to them in a language I did not understand.

I said, 'I would ask that you speak English, okay?'

He replied, 'Okay.'

So the Tactical police could tell who was exiting the house, I said, 'Can you tell me what you are wearing?'

He gave me these details and Goody passed them on to the Tactical team.

I said, 'This is what I want you to do. Firstly, prior to leaving the house you will pass the telephone to the next person. Do you understand that?'

'Yes.'

I said, 'Leave any weapons inside the house. Do you understand that?'

'No weapons.'

I said, 'You will place your hands on your head and walk straight out of the front door down the path. Do you understand that?'

'Yes.'

I said, 'You will keep walking very slowly until you are met by the police and follow their instructions. Do you understand that?'

'Yes.'

I said, 'Before you go, please repeat back to me what you have been told to do.'

He repeated the instructions. I confirmed with Goody that this man was ready to leave the house and he passed this on via the radio.

On receiving the go-ahead, I said, 'You can leave the house now. Please pass the phone to the next person.'

My instructions and conversation were being passed on to the Tactical team who had surrounded the unit. I could not see what was happening, I only had feedback from this team via Goody and the radio. I was told that the first man had left the townhouse and been arrested by the Tactical team without incident. From the information we had, this kidnapper had been incredibly forthcoming on the telephone and I didn't have a fight on my hands. In fact, once he opened the front door and saw one of the Tactical police, he became very compliant, doing exactly what I asked him to do.

I gave the other kidnappers the same instructions with the same results. I am still surprised that these very tough kidnappers allowed themselves to be arrested so easily and we didn't have a siege on our hands. However, once they looked at the heavily armed Tactical police, they must have realised just how outgunned they were.

These types of investigations use many police resources. In this case more than one hundred police were involved, including Local Area Command investigators, Major Crime Squad investigators, surveillance police, Police Airwing, State Protection Group Tactical Operations Unit and negotiators, technical police, Dog Squad, Crime Scene police, fingerprint police, and the Video Unit. It is such a relief and so satisfying when all these resources work together for a successful outcome: the return of the kidnapping victim, albeit very bruised, and six persons arrested and charged.

The boy's father Jim later wrote letters to the Commissioner of Police and the commander of the operation, thanking them for what they had done. He added, 'To Belinda and Goody, what can I say, you guys are just beautiful. Keep in touch, and here come the tears. Mark and Belinda, thanks.' When I found this letter years later I was the one who cried. This was such an emotionally charged situation and my feelings in knowing I had made such a difference to someone cannot be described in words.

I also had a chuckle at another part of Jim's letter, 'To the State Protection Group, guys, the back fence and compost bin will never be the same again, but who cares? You are all welcome back anytime to watch *Rambo*. But please leave the pump action shotguns and automatic weapons at the station. My neighbours have experienced enough action for this year.'

After all that, plus having very little sleep and working on the Hagland murder investigation at the same time, I was so looking forward to my day off, until my negotiator pager activated about 12.30pm. I was called out to a siege at Mt Druitt, a forty-five-minute high-speed drive for me. The situation took eight hours to resolve and I drove home to try and get some much-needed rest.

The following day, Monday 16 September, I was back on the Hagland murder investigation. It was time to interview suspects. At that stage the bugs we put in the Cushman house had confirmed Martin's involvement and contributed to Cushman's guilt in helping Martin flee the crime scene. This supported evidence from eyewitnesses to the assault.

I interviewed Sean Cushman, with his solicitor present, at the office of the Major Crime Squad South. In the meantime Aaron Martin, accompanied by his high-profile solicitor, presented himself to the officer in charge of the investigation, Detective Sergeant Adam Purcell at Bondi police station. Martin was charged with the murder of Brian Hagland. The next day I organised for blood and hair samples to be taken from Sean Cushman to confirm that he was not the person who had smeared blood in various places on the way to the Hagland assault. We also executed a search warrant at his home. On Wednesday 18 September I charged Sean Cushman with being an accessory after the fact of murder.

I was mentally and physically drained from the murder and kidnapping investigations. I needed some time out to recharge my batteries. I took four days off, then returned to work to put together the brief of evidence for the Hagland investigation with Detective Sergeant Purcell. This was a major and complex project, which involved organising all witness statements, the listening-device transcripts and police statements doing whatever follow-up work was necessary.

I spent the next few days on this and went on call again as a negotiator as well. On 26 September after finally finishing work at 5pm I headed home, had dinner and got ready to settle in for the evening. At about 8.30 my pager activated. A young man had barricaded himself in a house at Whalan, about forty-four kilometres west of Sydney, and threatened to commit suicide. It meant another forty-five-minute high-speed drive. I met the negotiation team near the house and spent the next fourteen hours with the other team members trying to convince the young man not to commit suicide.

By 11.30 the next morning the suicide intervention was over. To this day I cannot remember how the situation was resolved, whether the young man surrendered or whether it was a Tactical resolution, but he did not kill himself. I was bone tired, having been awake for more than twenty-eight hours, and I went home to get some well-deserved sleep.

On the morning of the following day I started work at Bondi police station to continue putting together the brief of evidence for Hagland. One of the Homicide supervisors rang me to say there had been a police shooting incident. A Critical Incident Investigation Team (CIIT) had been set up and I was required to attend as an investigator. I was worn out. I knew this would be a long and involved investigation but was told that no one else was available so I felt compelled to attend. The only way I could cope was to push all other thoughts out of my head and concentrate on this matter now at hand.

On 27 September two senior police, on their way to the church service for Police Remembrance Day, had come across a robbery at the Percy Marks jewellery store in Elizabeth Street in the city. There was a shootout between the police officers and armed robbers, one of whom was shot in the shoulder. The robbers escaped. Our role was to ascertain if the police officers had been justified in using their firearms.

I had never been involved in this type of investigation, but I knew the officer in charge, Detective Senior Sergeant Gordon, and was looking forward to working with him. After being briefed I headed out to the crime scene. Detective Senior Sergeant Gordon was extremely professional and easily took over from the local investigators to run the crime scene, ensuring it was set up properly.

We returned to the office, where another detective and I were to interview one of the police officers involved in the shooting. My work partner had never been part of this type of investigation either, but agreed to be in charge. I was glad he did; he would be required to put the brief of evidence together and I just didn't have the time to do that properly.

We conducted a lengthy interview with our senior police officer and given the evidence we had, were finally satisfied that he had used his firearm in accordance with the NSW police guidelines. Now we needed to interview the injured offender, but we did not have one; he had escaped in a getaway car with his accomplices. We did not know how seriously he was injured, although we had been told he had been shot in the shoulder, and we needed to find him quickly because of possible complications to his health. He had been hit with a controlled expansion projectile, otherwise known as a hollow point bullet, which is designed to expand on impact due to the hollowed-out pit in the tip. This causes more tissue damage than an ordinary bullet and can lead to greater blood loss.

The hunt for the armed robbers went on for hours, to no avail. I finally finished at midnight after another sixteen-hour shift. Once again I was looking forward to my free weekend, hoping for a quiet time as a negotiator. Sometimes I had been on call for a week without one negotiator callout, so I hoped the weekend would be uninterrupted.

Famous last words. On Saturday 28 September the negotiator pager activated about 11am. At least I had had a decent night's sleep. This time I was summoned to the Windsor area to meet our negotiator team leader and the Tactical police and try to arrest an escaped prisoner safely. This prisoner was extremely volatile with a lengthy history of armed robberies and other offences involving weapons and violence. The Tactical police were to arrest him during a high-risk vehicle stop and we negotiators were to stay at a safe distance, only becoming involved if a siege developed. So I was on standby for most of the day. Eventually the escaped prisoner was safely apprehended and I finished at 6pm. So much for my relaxing day off.

About 8.30pm my pager activated again. This time, a man had taken a woman hostage at Crows Nest. I was instantly alert, aided by a rush of adrenalin. It was raining heavily when I arrived at the house in Ernest Street and the Tactical team were already there, as was Whitey, the primary negotiator. The rest of our negotiation team hadn't arrived at this stage. We were told that the hostage, Grace, had tried to end her three-month relationship with Ivan Christov earlier that day. Christov, armed with a small open flick knife, had confronted her and her mother in the bedroom of her home. He punched Grace and dragged her into the kitchen, where he grabbed a thirty-centimetre carving knife. He then dragged her back to the bedroom and barricaded himself and Grace in there, threatening to kill her.

One of the uniform officers had climbed over the police barricade and was in the bedroom trying to negotiate with Christov. Christov was becoming more aggressive and the emotion in the room was intensifying and threatening to get out of control. Our first job was to try and calm the situation by getting the police officer out of the room without jeopardising either his safety or Grace's. We needed to do this before the police officer became another hostage or Christov stabbed Grace.

The Tactical team gave Whitey and me a ballistic vest each. This had ceramic high velocity trauma plates, front and back, and weighed about twenty kilograms. I simply couldn't get it over my head due to its awkward size and weight and needed the help of the Tactical police. I would spend the next eight hours on my feet and wearing this vest.

My role as the secondary negotiator was to back up Whitey, giving him support and relieve him if necessary. We knew what we had to do and we needed to do it fast. There was no time to sit around discussing our roles and gathering more intelligence. Years of training and experience were about to be put into practice.

We went through the front door of the house into a hallway. The first room to the right was the bedroom in which Christov, Grace and the young uniformed police officer were holed up. The top panel of the bedroom door was missing and the bottom still intact, and I saw that Christov had set up barricades. The bed had been overturned and the wire frame was against the doorway. A heavy-looking wardrobe, a number of boxes and other furniture had been stacked up around the doorway, making a quick entry into the room impossible. The mattress had been placed against the front external window, blocking any view into the room.

Inside the room we were confronted with a very tense situation. Christov, wild-eyed and crazy-haired, was shouting that he would kill his hostage if the young police officer did not get out of the bedroom. He was holding Grace in a headlock with the carving knife pressed against one side of her neck and the pocketknife pressed against the other. Grace was screaming for help, her white top covered in blood where Christov had already cut her neck. She also had injuries to her hand and deep cuts to her thigh. The young uniformed officer was pleading with Christov to put down the knife.

The presence of the uniformed cop, with all good intention to rescue Grace, was only serving to worsen what was already a very dangerous situation. There was no chance he could get close enough to disarm Ivan before Ivan had the chance to run both knives though Grace's neck.

Whitey quickly introduced himself to Christov as a police negotiator.

Then in a clear, calm voice he said, 'I would like you to let the police officer out of the room, please.'

He needed to repeat himself a number of times as Christov's fury was entirely focused on the young officer. Whitey turned to the police officer and told him to back very slowly past the barricade and out of the room. The young officer had a look of disbelief on his face; he didn't want to leave the victim in the hands of this madman, and I didn't blame him. I also felt for Grace in her helplessness, being left alone in the bedroom with Christov. She saw her only security leave the room, and she would not have understood why. Christov's rage was intensifying and it looked as if he was ready to torture her further or kill her. She was in grave danger.

As soon as the young police officer climbed over the last obstacle and left the room, Whitey started talking to Christov. At this stage I noticed that Christov had set up mirrors that enabled him to see a short way along the hallway. It was a very cunning move, as he would have time to kill Grace if he saw anyone coming towards the room.

Over the next few hours Whitey spoke with Christov. Sometimes Christov would lose his temper, shout that he was going to kill Grace and make what appeared to be small, superficial cuts in her neck while she screamed for help. I asked ambulance officers whether these cuts could be life-threatening, but they said they were not and gave me instructions, which we would later pass on to Christov, about how to treat the cuts. The information from the ambulance officers was crucial; Christov could kill Grace in seconds. We believed he would certainly do that if he knew Tactical police intended to charge into the bedroom, as they would take more than a few seconds to disarm him. Even if Tactical police had been able to shoot Christov, he could have had time to kill Grace. Negotiation appeared to be the only option at that point. It was a very difficult situation, made worse by the look of sheer terror on Grace's tear-stained face.

Initially we had received virtually no information about Christov, and finding out more was crucial in planning our negotiation strategy. When we realised we were in for the long haul, our consulting psychiatrist arrived.

During the course of a very tense high-risk negotiation like this, it is imperative that the team has time out for briefings. During one of Whitey's conversations he told Christov that we intended to leave the bedroom doorway for a short time.

Christov said, 'If you leave the doorway clear I will lay her on the floor and hold the carving knife against her like this.' He pointed the tip of the carving knife at Grace's chest, over her heart.

'I will lie on top of her with the knife in between us and if anyone enters the room I will let go.' He would drop his weight onto the carving knife, forcing it into her chest. Grace naturally became very distressed, which only aggravated Christov. Because she was in such danger Whitey and I decided very quickly that I would remain at the doorway while Whitey was briefed.

I noticed Christov becoming more agitated with Grace's crying and suggested that she might be allowed to change her shirt. It looked cold and wet, covered in blood, and this might also have been upsetting her. He agreed and allowed her to change her top, picking out another among the clothes strewn on the floor.

At another stage Christov said, 'I just want to get my cigarettes. They are in that bag,' pointing to a bag near the bedroom door.

'Sure,' I said.

I had no problem with that and I raised my hands slightly, palms turned towards Christov to show there would be no trouble. I knew that there was no way the Tactical guys could get over the barrier to grab Christov, or possibly fire a shot, before he got back to Grace. I was so focused on the situation in the bedroom that when Christov moved slightly towards the doorway I took an involuntary step back, still with my hands in the air.

In my peripheral vision, I noticed movements on either side of me in the hallway. Two Tactical teams, who had been watching me, had raised their Heckler and Koch MP5 9mm sub-machine guns in anticipation of a possible assault or surrender. I could see them both advancing, their guns at the ready, thinking that something was about to happen. I was so focused that I hadn't even realised they were there. I also saw that Whitey had come to the top of the hallway. As both my hands were already raised I turned my palms out and gave a slight shake of my head to let the Tactical guys know to stop where they were. They understood the message and backed off. Christov retrieved the cigarettes and moved back to his position, thankfully unaware of what had been happening in the hallway.

I felt totally helpless in not being able to do more for Grace. I saw that she was scared and in pain, but I could only watch.

I couldn't be seen by Christov to give her too much attention or offer her comfort, for fear he would hurt her again just to taunt us.

Whitey came back to the doorway soon after and I left to have a break and be briefed. I was told that Christov had a lengthy criminal history involving violence, particularly against women, as well as other offences. In 1975, at the age of twenty-four he had been charged with attempted murder and a number of assaults, one involving firearms after being rejected by a woman he had been involved with.

The negotiations continued over eight hours. No matter how tense it became or how much Christov threatened Grace, Whitey's voice was always calm and reassuring. I don't know how Whitey was feeling physically at that point but my back was killing me from standing up in the ballistic vest.

Christov would at times speak to Grace in a Slavic language so an interpreter was called in. At other times he would yell at Grace that the police were going to kill him. Christov was given coffee at his request and occasionally we watched him snort white powder up his nose. He told us this was cocaine to keep him awake.

At a time when he was calm Whitey told him how to treat Grace's wounds, telling him this would be looked on favourably when he came out. It was considered a good sign if we could get him to look after his hostage.

Whitey kept asking Christov to hand over the knives, to allow Grace to leave and to come out of the bedroom, but Christov refused. He asked for his solicitor to come to the house, but we thought that would be too dangerous. Christov was unstable and we couldn't predict what he would do. There was no problem allowing him access to his solicitor at the police station but not here. We compromised and organised for his solicitor to record a message telling Christov he would be waiting for him at North Sydney police station, further reassurance to Christov that he would be coming out.

About 4.20am, nearly eight hours after our initial callout, Christov allowed Grace to hand Whitey the large carving knife. We felt a breakthrough had been made at last, but still we could not let our guard down. Christov still had Grace and the smaller knife. Whitey asked for the smaller pocket knife, and without warning, perhaps as a final act of opposition, Christov threw the pocketknife straight at him. Fortunately Whitey was wearing the ballistic vest and the knife glanced off his chest.

We finally had both knives but we could not arrest Christov. He could have used other objects in the room to injure Grace, and we did not know whether he had any concealed weapons. At least he was showing a serious commitment to ending the siege peacefully.

After more negotiation Christov finally allowed Grace to leave the room. As soon as she came out she was put into the care of the ambulance officers because she had some serious injuries; deep stab wounds to her thighs, severe cuts on her hand where she had tried to defend herself initially, lacerations to her abdomen, and superficial wounds on her neck. She was also suffering from shock.

We could not relax; now was the time to change our focus. We had been concentrating on achieving Grace's release, but now the issue was whether Christov would feel he had lost control and had no hope. Would he become suicidal? Our role as negotiators was about saving lives, in this case not just that of the hostage but also that of the hostage taker.

Whitey and I only had a few minutes to discuss this while Grace was leaving the bedroom, but it was enough for Whitey to refocus his thinking around possible suicide intervention. He eventually managed to coax Christov from the room. Christov was arrested by the Tactical police and taken to North Sydney police station to see his solicitor.

Whitey and I were not involved in the interview and charging process; our part had ended. We all went back to North Sydney to have an operational debriefing with the Tactical police. Later we heard that a makeshift bed had been set up in the roof of the house directly above Grace's bedroom; a blanket, doona and some McDonald's wrappers were found. Whilst investigators initially believed Christov had done this, it was in fact the work of the Tactical police, who had been ready to go through the ceiling if necessary.

I finished at 7am on Sunday morning 29 September. I was shattered, having in the previous forty-eight hours been involved in a police shooting investigation and two negotiator callouts, the second of which was one of the most mentally and physically exhausting negotiations I had ever experienced. It had been a long few days, as well as a very busy month. I went straight to bed and fell into a dead sleep.

About 8.30pm that night my pager activated yet again. This time I was to negotiate with a woman armed with a knife and again this was on the north side of Sydney. When I arrived about forty-five minutes later I could see that the other negotiators all looked as tired as I felt. None of us could believe the week we were having. Fortunately, the woman surrendered herself after a short negotiation and we finished at 11pm.

September was almost over. It was time to return the negotiator pager, take the home phone off the hook, enjoy a few well-earned days off and reintroduce myself to my husband. It had never occurred to me that I might have been taking

on too much; working both Homicide and high-risk negotiation. The reality was, as the month of September showed, that
I was becoming too subjective and not able to think objec-
tively in terms of my own welfare. My approach to work was
almost paramilitary: I had an overwhelming sense of duty
that allowed me to disassociate and tolerate the hours and the
situations I was involved with. I was almost like a gambler
at the casino, without external references to or knowledge
about whether it was night or day, just this disconnection
allowing me to concentrate on the job at hand.

I felt as if the work I was doing as a negotiator effectively
kept me going through what was a particularly dark and busy
time at the Homicide Unit, the balance of light and dark, saving lives versus death. To me, one balanced the other and I
needed to know there was a positive to offset the images of
death surrounding me.

Many years later, when I no longer had work to keep me
busy, the images of the distress in Grace's face, her bloodstained shirt and my feeling of utter helplessness as she was
being stabbed would come flooding back. I had not given
myself the chance to process any of these awful images and
they were now building up in my internal image library. This
would eventually take its toll.

CHAPTER

10

Par for the course

Over the next few months I was called to attend various negotiator situations and assisted at a negotiators' course at Goulburn Police Academy. Helping out as a role player for the practical exercises on the course was a form of training in itself. I could be asked to play a depressed or suicidal person, an armed offender, a hostage or hostage taker. Psychiatrists advised us how to carry out the role with information about the behaviour and expectations of people in these situations. Later, when attending various callouts, I had a better appreciation of the fears, anger, loneliness and sadness they might be feeling. Showing compassion that is genuine is a key ingredient to establishing rapport. Secondly, and very importantly, by playing these roles and speaking with trainee police negotiators I could still learn positive things to say and what not to say during negotiations, and learn from the trainees' mistakes.

In late 1996 I was selected to undergo a two-week accelerated mediation training course with the Community Justice Centre (CJC). Funded by the NSW government, the CJC provides free mediation to help resolve disputes ranging from family issues to neighbour disputes and conflicts in the workplace. The last time negotiators were invited to participate in this course had been in 1988, so I felt fortunate to be involved.

The intention of this course was to complement our negotiator training, as mediation is a different way of resolving conflict. Negotiation is very focused on actively finding solutions with the other party, including using skills to influence the thinking and behaviour of others. The negotiator is a problem solver. The mediator, on the other hand, is a facilitator. Mediation involves exploring perceptions and acknowledging emotions, which can sometimes assist with psychological release. It focuses on the necessity for the other parties to identify the issues, develop options and make decisions themselves, the principle being that anyone involved in the decision making is more likely to stay with the outcome, rather than having a solution imposed.

In 1996 I started a Graduate Certificate in Dispute Resolution, which included negotiation, crisis negotiation and advanced mediation. This complemented the CJC mediation training. I found the principles of mediation, including having a person take ownership for bringing about a solution, another tool I could use in my work. I had the opportunity to put the CJC training and my course into practice in January 1997.

About 7.30am on the morning of Friday 17th I was called out as a negotiator to a suicide intervention at Lighthouse

Reserve, Vaucluse. I was on standby for court this day so was wearing a very smart navy dress, pearls and shoes. Not particularly suitable attire for a negotiator callout, but I felt I would only be there for a couple of hours to assist the team until I was called to attend court. At that stage there were only two negotiators and the Police Rescue Squad.

I saw a man sitting on the wrong side of the fence near the edge of the cliff, facing out to sea. We did not know who he was or why he was there at that stage. My offsider Megan introduced herself and starting talking to the man while I retained the role of team leader. For the next couple of hours it was a one-sided conversation. The man didn't even turn his head to look at us but remained sitting on the ledge, staring out towards the sea. I could now see that this was going to be a lengthy negotiation, so we called in the rest of the team.

For five hours we alternated between negotiators to talk with the man, in the hope that one of us would establish a connection with him. My court matter had been adjourned so I could also try to talk to the man, and again it was a one-sided conversation. It was too dangerous a situation for Rescue Squad police to go over the fence with a safety harness; as the man was sitting right on the ledge and might jump before they could get to him.

Even though he wouldn't speak to us, at least he was still alive. However, one of our consulting psychiatrists told the negotiating team to start mentally preparing for the worst. The information we now had about our man made the situation even more dangerous. His name was John and he was a systems analyst who worked for a government department and was heavily involved with Australia's defence system. He had made a mistake at work involving various components within our defence system, and felt the only way out was to commit suicide by throwing himself off the cliff. At the same time, he was also the only person who could fix the problem.

Over the next few hours we were able to get some information from John, but the negotiations were still very one-sided. We were able to place food and water over the fence, making sure he knew we were not going to try and seize him. To provide him with food and water was important. It was a hot summer's day and we were concerned that he might become dehydrated, faint, or lose the ability to properly concentrate and thus make a reckless decision to end his life.

Fortunately one of John's work superiors arrived. We did not tell John this as we were unsure of his reaction and we didn't want to risk upsetting him. This superior not only wanted John back at work but was prepared to do everything in his power to get him any help he needed as he was a highly valued worker. This was fantastic news to us and definitely information we could use in our negotiations.

While the advice from the psychiatrist had been to prepare for him to jump I still felt positive that while he was still sitting on that ledge we had a chance. We decided I should get closer to him, making it easier to talk to him rather than being a face calling out from behind the fence. I needed to wear the safety harness to go over the fence, which would not have worked with the dress I was wearing, so I borrowed a pair of grey overalls from one of our technical police.

It took careful negotiation just to let John know I was coming over the fence with another bottle of water so he wouldn't be spooked, think I was trying to rescue him, and jump. I made it very clear I was going to sit on one of the rocks near him, just out of arm's reach.

I might add here I do not like heights, not one bit. Every year on the negotiator's course the commander organises a climb over the Harbour Bridge for new negotiators to get used to heights and the Bridge in case they are called out to a suicide intervention there. Luckily for me this was brought in after I completed the three-year negotiator course, and I respectfully declined or became scarce whenever the subject came up.

As I climbed the fence I continued reassuring John about what I was doing so he would not become agitated. I could now clearly see he was sitting on a rock right at the edge of the cliff, his legs hanging over. I think that once he saw the fear in my face he realised I was speaking the truth and was happy for me to stay close but just out of reach. I could now have a more intimate conversation with him, with more chance to ascertain his emotions and explore his thinking.

We sat and talked for some time. I could see that John appeared very embarrassed by his situation, being proud of his professionalism at work but so humiliated about his mistake that he could see no way out but to commit suicide. This was a perfect situation for the use of mediation techniques, as John needed to be involved in solving the problem for himself. He had to make a decision and he would certainly not be coerced into it. I reflected back to John the important points he made and asked him questions intended to explore his own emotions and feelings.

Finally John decided to come back from the edge of the cliff to try and resolve his situation. I was almost caught off guard as I had expected to be sitting on that rock for a lot longer. However, he was still in a very precarious position, seated on a rock on a very small cliff ledge with his legs hanging over the cliff face. He had been sitting there for some time so I was watching him intently as we both went to stand up. At this point I was still out of arm's reach as the rope for the safety harness was still tied off on the fence.

Then John tripped. The bottle of water I had given him had been just near his feet and he must have knocked it and trodden on it when he stood up.

It felt like slow motion. He was so close to the edge I automatically put my arm out and went for him but the rope and safety harness stopped me. I was simply too far away. In my mind's eye I saw him go over the edge ...

I still don't know how he did it, but he was able to steady himself. We looked at each other and both knew how close he had come to 'accidentally' falling off the edge of the cliff face. We then walked back to the fence together and he climbed over it to safe ground. Shortly after, he was taken to the local hospital for a psychiatric evaluation.

The team was elated at the result, especially after we had been mentally preparing ourselves for the prospect that he would commit suicide in front of us. I still don't believe there is really any way to prepare yourself for seeing that, except perhaps treating the psychological after-effects. I believe that even if you do everything possible to prevent it, if someone really wants to end their life, they will.

This mentally exhausting negotiation lasted about ten hours. I later found that the top of my back was blistered from exposure to the sun. My concentration had been such that I hadn't even noticed that my skin was burning and certainly hadn't thought to ask for sunscreen.

In 1995 the head of the Hostage Negotiation Unit, Israeli Police Commander Eli Landau, visited Australia and took part in a number of NSW training courses and lectures.

Mr Landau, who had travelled all over the world in the study of hostage negotiation, stated, 'Although you may not have the experience with terrorists, I think the way Australian Police negotiation is organised and run is the best in the world.' For someone so experienced in counter-terrorism to give such high commendation is testament to the experience of the trainers and training programs run not only in NSW but Australia-wide.

In December 1996 I was selected to attend a counter-terrorist negotiator course run by the Standing Advisory Committee on Commonwealth/State Cooperation for Protection Against Violence (SAC-PAV). This was established after the Hilton Hotel bombing in 1978, providing a formal mechanism to develop responses to terrorism. The course was hosted by the Victorian Police and was held in Melbourne. Invitations were extended to each of the police forces in Australia, and sixteen participants would be selected. Goody, my negotiation team leader, was the other participant from NSW.

We were to fly to Melbourne on 8 December and return on the 14th. However, in the meantime I found out I had to give evidence at the committal proceedings of Graham Mailes for the murder of Kim Meredith. If I had to go to Albury during the week of the course, I wouldn't be allowed to start it. Fortunately I gave my evidence on Friday 6 December and spent Saturday driving the 570 kilometres home to pack and fly to Melbourne on Sunday.

I was finally at the airport ready to depart. I put my bag on the conveyor belt to go through the security check and walked through the metal detector. As I went to pick up my bag a security guard stopped me.

'Excuse me, ma'am. Do you have any bullets in your bag?'

What? I thought. I was mortified.

I quickly said, 'I'm a police officer,' in case he thought I was a potential armed offender and decided to arrest me on the spot. 'I must have left them in there when I was packing.'

He took a look at my police identification and I saw him glance behind me. I think my companions had also acted very quickly, also producing their police identification badges. I was very embarrassed but quickly checked my bag. Yes there was a 'speed strip' containing five .38 calibre bullets, which would have been very obvious on the security screen.

So here I was off to a counter-terrorist course carrying hollow point bullets onto a plane. Not a good look. Fortunately this was before 9/11, otherwise I am sure I would have been arrested first and asked questions later.

The problem now, apart from embarrassing myself in front of the commander, was what to do with the bullets. I could not throw them away, and I couldn't take them with me. Fortunately one of my colleagues wives offered to take them home with her.

The counter-terrorist negotiators' course is aimed at developing the negotiation skills necessary for handling prolonged and complex international terrorist incidents. CT negotiators negotiate on behalf of the prime minister or state premier and on behalf of state governments when there is a terrorist incident. In normal domestic situations, police negotiate on behalf of the Commissioner of Police.

An Australian Security Intelligence Organisation (ASIO) representative spoke about current potential threats; Stephen Romano, an international consultant from the FBI, discussed the lessons learned from the Waco (1993) and Freeman (1996) sieges. (The Waco siege had occurred after a shootout between the US Bureau of Alcohol, Tobacco, and Firearms

(ATF) and members of a religious cult when the ATF tried to arrest their leader, David Koresh, and senior members on firearms warrants. A fifty-one-day siege ensued with the FBI. A tactical assault with CS gas was authorised and during the raid it is believed that cult members set fire to the compound, resulting in the deaths of seventy-six people. The Freeman siege involved a group who believed they were a law unto themselves. A siege developed after the FBI went to execute arrest warrants. After an eighty-one-day siege sixteen people surrendered peacefully.) There were also lectures on the current Australian government counter-terrorism policy, negotiation team management and strategy development. We received instruction on the differences between domestic and counter-terrorist negotiations and between criminal hostage takers and terrorists. Terrorists have a political agenda, not a personal one, and may be prepared to risk their lives, and terrorist hostage incidents are by their political nature very complex.

We were divided into groups and given a terrorist-hostage-taking scenario with various instructions that we would brainstorm. These included preparing opening statements for the primary negotiator; developing strategies for responding to questioning by the hostage taker over initial demands; discussing issues or problems that might face negotiators and identifying resources available to negotiators. We would then present our findings to the class.

We then had a two-day terrorist-hostage-taking practical exercise where we were divided into negotiating teams of four people, each taking it in turns to be the primary negotiator. It was a very psychologically demanding and realistic exercise. Initially I was quite nervous. Not only was I going to have to use all my negotiating and communication skills, but

I was being observed and evaluated as a future CT negotiator. There was also some professional interstate rivalry and I did not want to let the NSW side down. As time went on I became too focussed to worry about nerves, intent on listening to the terrorist to ensure I heard and interpreted his views, his thoughts, his emotions and his demands, as well as gathering as much intelligence as possible. I was trying to think one step ahead, being prepared with appropriate responses, and carrying out my own strategies and advice from the negotiation team. It was an exhausting course altogether, and I was very glad to see the end of the two-day exercise.

Under the auspices of SACPAV, in line with Australia's antiterrorist arrangements, there are two major National Anti-Terrorist Exercises (NATEX) held each year. Participants in these counter-terrorist exercises are a multi-agency group, including police, fire and rescue, ambulance, Australian Federal Police, ASIO, Australian Defence Force and government ministers. These exercises are vital to maintain and continually hone the skills of those involved.

At the beginning of August 1997 I was involved in a SACPAV exercise in Adelaide, where I was to play the role of a terrorist. There were at least three of us who were role-playing as terrorists with a number of hostages. I knew we would be in the stronghold for two to three days so had packed clothes and extra food accordingly. We were based on a property with a number of buildings and only one road leading in, otherwise we were surrounded by water. By blocking the entrance to that road we were effectively cut off and on our own little island.

We 'terrorists' took the hostages, firing shots to injure or kill various persons, and barricaded ourselves on the island. I was interested to see how the time factor worked: the time taken by Tactical police to organise their equipment and cover the perimeters, and for CT negotiators to get enough information to make a telephone call to us, was much longer than we had anticipated. Over the next two days, at all hours, each terrorist spoke with CT negotiators by phone. We had a separate telephone in the stronghold used to relay messages between the exercise organisers and ourselves. Sometimes the exercise organisers told us to apply pressure on the CT negotiators during the course of negotiations, at other times they told us to test the surveillance teams, including both the Tactical police units and the Australian Defence Force. On these occasions we might be asked to go for a walk outside the compound to see if the surveillance teams could detect anything.

I found playing the role of a terrorist an amazing learning experience. By the second evening, after very little sleep and no shower, I was looking forward to seeing how the exercise would be resolved, knowing I would finally be seeing Australia's elite Special Air Service (SAS) in action. Prior to their arrival we had instructors come into the stronghold and place us in various rooms, some terrorists in rooms with hostages, a terrorist by himself, and hostages by themselves. I was in a room with another terrorist and a hostage. All us terrorists were armed with fake rifles and various firearms.

And then we heard the Black Hawks. We had been given a few pairs of night-vision goggles so we could see the descent of the Black Hawk helicopters and the SAS operatives. Watching them come in for an assault under the cover of darkness was absolutely amazing; they are an extraordinarily professional unit.

The room I was in was pitch black, no light on. I could feel the anticipation of the forthcoming assault, this was

Australia's elite fighting force and considered one of the best in the world, and I was on the receiving end, holding a fake rifle.

I did not have to wait for long. There was an almighty bang as the door was kicked open. I aimed my rifle towards two black figures, saw some flashes and I knew I had been shot with paintball. In a few seconds it was all over for my terrorist mate and me.

A debriefing was held for the SAS operatives before they exited the stronghold and back to the Black Hawks. We were also picked up and transported back to the South Australian Police Academy for a quick debrief and finally a hot shower.

I found the NATEX a remarkable learning experience for a negotiator, and I would have to be honest and say the high point was the opportunity to watch the SAS at work.

CHAPTER

11

Extortion

May 1997 started out as a busy month. I had two on-call periods as a negotiator and the committal hearing into the Hagland murder had begun; both Cushman and Martin were committed for trial to the Supreme Court. Aaron Martin was later found guilty of the lesser charge of maliciously inflicting grievous bodily harm with intent. He received a sentence of five years in prison, minimum term two years and three months. The Hagland family and Connie Casey were devastated. Sean Cushman was also found guilty to being an accessory. He was given a good behaviour bond for five years. Considering Martin's previous violent history, including punching and kicking another person under similar circumstances, I was disgusted at the sentence Martin was given.

On Thursday 22 May my negotiation team leader rang me about an extortion demand at one of Australia's major food companies, also one of the world's largest. About 10am I went into the company's head office in the city and met with investigators from Major Crime Squad South. The investigation had been codenamed Operation Billiat. A two-page typed letter delivered by courier contained a demand for over $4 million, the largest extortion demand ever made in Australia. The ransom was to be paid the following day, otherwise various products in stores throughout Australia would be contaminated. An additional $1 million per week would be required until the ransom was paid or the company had to permanently close in Australia. The extortionist wrote that 'success in poisoning people was not considered essential' but 'turning people away from' the company's products was the real issue. The extortionist allowed for police to be contacted if the company so wished but an additional $1 million would be added to the demand if police intervened. If he agreed to payment of the extortion demand, the CEO was told to place an advertisement in the *Sydney Morning Herald* Lost and Found section, the wording of which was provided in the letter.

The extortionist had already directed company staff, via a faxed document, to a large retail grocery store where a jar of instant coffee had been contaminated. Company staff were able to quickly take all the coffee jars off the shelf. One had a small puncture mark in the paper membrane, which was proof, the company staff said, that it had been tampered with. This contaminated jar was kept as evidence and retained by police for further analysis. The contaminate was later found to be a form of insecticide which could induce sickness and possibly cause a person to lapse into unconsciousness and even death.

The company's crisis management team, comprising senior management, risk-management consultants flown in from

Melbourne and police investigators, were pulling out all stops to try and identify the extortionist. The company would sustain significant financial loss, millions of dollars, if all food products needed to be recalled, as well as further financial losses every day the products were not available to the public. Analysis of the coffee and jar was fast tracked, staff at the newsagent from where the fax had been sent were interviewed, as were employees of the courier service. A description of a man was given.

The extortionist had addressed the mail to the CEO by name and had telephoned his secretary to confirm that the CEO had received the fax. On the premise that the extortionist might get in touch again, my role was to provide simple negotiation strategies for the CEO and his secretary, including the development of suggested dialogue with the extortionist. Even though both were under immense pressure they were very receptive.

It was decided to place the advertisement in the newspaper as requested. Unfortunately it would not be published until the following day, Friday 23 May. This was the deadline for payment, even though no account details had been provided.

About 3.25pm one of the company managers came into the meeting room with a two-page fax from the extortionist. This time a twin pack of a particular brand of yoghurt had been contaminated, and the fax gave details of the store and suburb. Store management were immediately contacted and detectives were dispatched. Later that afternoon they returned to the head office with fifteen twin packs of the yoghurt, one tub of which had a small tear in the foil lid. Even so, the presence of a contaminate could not be confirmed.

The immediate problem was the risk to the general public if the contaminated yoghurt had already been sold. If we couldn't confirm that we had the tub of contaminated yoghurt, a product recall notice would need to be issued urgently. This was something the company naturally did not want to happen.

After much discussion, it was decided to open each tub of yoghurt and smell it for the presence of a contaminate. No distinct smell was noticed. The CEO wished to stir the yoghurt with a spoon to see if that would produce a smell. The investigators agreed on condition that a separate spoon was used for each tub of yoghurt, thereby preserving the integrity of the exhibits. A packet of clean plastic spoons was found and a clean spoon placed in each tub. Every tub of yoghurt was stirred then smelled but still no distinctive odour could be detected.

Due to the very serious possibility that an unsuspecting customer might have purchased the product, the company quickly issued a press release advising that the particular yoghurt from that store was not fit for consumption and should be returned. The next day was the day the extortionist had demanded payment. I arrived at the company head office about 7am. After being briefed by the police investigation team I sat down with the CEO and later his secretary to go through negotiation strategies should the extortionist ring them personally. During the day I was involved in a number of meetings with the crisis management team and the police investigators to discuss various long- and short-term strategies should the extortion continue, otherwise it was a waiting game.

About 3pm the extortionist sent another fax to the CEO, this time from a newsagent in Victoria. The extortionist had obviously seen the advertisement and the fax was headed 'Agreement noted' with instructions about payment, including bank account details. The extortionist added 'as a courtesy you will be spared the third treasure hunt'. The hunt now escalated, with further meetings, enquiries about the newsagent and further conversations about negotiation with the CEO and his secretary. I finished about eleven that night with no further word from the extortionist.

Over the weekend a team of NSW police investigators travelled to Victoria to work with the Victorian Police Special Response Group. A special fraud alert was placed on the bank account, a business account opened at a Victorian branch the previous week. All documents relevant to the account were seized. Information was taken from the bank tellers who had set up this bank account, which was in the name of Greg Butcher. This man had told one of the tellers that he was an ex-policeman. Inquiries were made about the birth certificate and company documents he presented, including personal references.

The following week, from Monday 26 to Friday 30 May, one team of investigators worked from Melbourne and the other team and I remained with the company's head office in case of further contact with the extortionist. By this stage the company's crisis-management team had flown out a risk consultant from their insurance company in London. Every morning I spoke with the CEO and his secretary about negotiating strategies and contingencies, then had to leave as I was running a drug trial at the Sydney District Court. Every afternoon I would check back to see how the extortion investigation was progressing. I also had a number of discussions with my negotiation team leader in Melbourne. The combined NSW/Victoria investigators in Melbourne were starting to close in on the extortionist – we just needed some additional evidence.

It was interesting being involved with the company's crisis-management team at this stage. At one point the insurance company representative from London wanted the bank teller to be given a list of instructions and questions to ask the extortionist when he came in to the branch – he had not finalised all paperwork when he opened the account, and needed to do so before he could make a withdrawal. This idea had merit but there were some rudimentary problems. We told the insurance man that things were better kept simple. It was a small branch of the bank, we didn't know whether the extortionist knew the inner workings of the branch and the staff; the bank teller was already under pressure and being told to use a police listening device and a lawful telephone intercept. We advised it would be better if the teller only asked some very basic things about which she was confident rather than have her become nervous and alert the extortionist. We did not want to risk him getting wind of the police operation and we couldn't use undercover police officers.

On Monday 26 May the combined police investigation team in Victoria had a breakthrough. A man had gone to a branch in Victoria and tried to withdraw $10,000 from the business account without providing any identification. He told the branch manager that his wallet had just been stolen at the markets. He also said he was expecting four million dollars to be paid into the account. The branch manager had told him that most third-party deposits were not processed immediately and he should check with the company to see when they made the deposit and where. The man had left the bank saying he would go and make those inquiries. The bank teller recognised the business account as the same one she and her branch manager had dealt with on the previous Friday afternoon.

On Monday 26 May a man rang the bank's customer service centre and asked for a balance on the business account. When he was asked for a password he said he didn't have one. The customer service officer noted that the account appeared to show warnings about possible fraud, but no telephone number for their fraud department appeared and the man was told how to go about getting a password on his account. He asked the customer service officer whether any money had been paid into the account, saying he was setting up a small business. The customer service officer told him the information on the account was confidential.

About 2pm the following day a man telephoned the original bank, identified himself as Greg Butcher and spoke with the bank teller, who quickly activated the telephone intercept. He asked about withdrawing money from other branches and whether any money had been deposited into the account, and was told that it now had a substantial balance. The bank teller said she needed to see his original birth certificate to verify his identification, and Greg Butcher said he would provide that soon.

Police surveillance continued to be carried out on this branch of the bank while other investigators were checking birth certificates and business records. They examined a great number of documents.

On the Thursday came the breakthrough evidence we needed; a telephone number that seemed to be unintentionally written on two separate business registration documents. The description of the person lodging these documents was also similar to those given by the other witnesses. This telephone number could have been a red herring but luck and some very good police work by the joint NSW/Victorian teams gave us this lead.

It was the home number belonging to the ex-wife of a man named Matthew Mills. She told police that their marriage had broken down some months earlier and Matthew had been made redundant from his job in April. Her description of Matthew tallied with the one the bank tellers had given. She also gave police his current Melbourne address. A few days later when she was formally interviewed she added that Matthew had told her he was going to Sydney for a few days as he wanted time away to think about things. She said that a few years previously both she and Matthew had decided to boycott the company's products, taking a moral stand because of negative publicity about the company's business practices.

The following day Victorian investigators interviewed Matthew Mills at his home address. This conversation was lawfully recorded. Matthew Mills's voice on tape appeared to be the same as that of Greg Butcher, recorded when he was talking to the teller. Mills was put under twenty-four-hour surveillance.

On Sunday 1 June my negotiation team leader told me the investigators needed more assistance in Melbourne. Being familiar with the case, I flew down the next day to change roles from negotiator to investigator.

On Monday 2 June a police officer came forward and said he knew Matthew Mills. He had met him some years earlier through a mutual friend and saw him socially. He knew Mills had travelled to Sydney and believed he returned on 23 May. He had been told Mills had made the trip to 'clear his mind' because he was getting a divorce and had been retrenched. This police officer said the previous year Mills had asked whether the record of his fingerprints taken when he was a police officer could be returned to him. He had told Mills he could write in to the Police Department to have the record destroyed. This police officer confirmed that the voice of Greg Butcher and Matthew Mills were one and the same. Victorian police confirmed that Mills was indeed a former police officer and had requested his fingerprints be destroyed as recently as the previous month.

Police were closing in on Matthew Mills and a search warrant for his home was issued. He was arrested just before 6pm on the evening of 2 June.

Mills gave police a number of folders from his backpack – the total of his assistance in the investigation. They contained information about the business bank account he had opened.

Of the documents he gave to police, one was a letter that read:

> [The name of the company in Sydney] have been chosen because of
> 1. As a large distributor of food items they are extremely vulnerable
> 2. They are large enough to extort significant moneys from
> 3. They already have a significant proportion of disillusioned customers due to the two previous [company name] boycotts by impact which would be readily mobilised against them in an anti-media campaign.

The next heading of the letter was 'Essentially the crime works like this' followed by:

> 1. some food stocks are poisoned;
> 2. a letter is sent advising them of the poisoning, demanding money
> 3. if [company name] pay then poisoning stops

   4. if [company name] don't pay then the poisonings con-
      tinue and increase demands until they give in.

The next heading 'To do':

   Develop an extortion letter
   Find out details
   Leave a message in the personal section of designated
      paper
   Sort out safe laundry details
   Get the name and number of the CEO's secretary
   Get details of Sydney delivery service
   Do a letter and do initial fax
   Get Melbourne, Sydney and Adelaide paper details for
      lodgement times

The next heading 'Notes':

   Don't leave fingerprints on anything, whether a caravan,
      rubbish, letter, poison stock, etcetera
   Chosen items are (Company brand) coffee jars, tube of
      condensed milk
   Don't use alcohol wipe cloths
   Use a reverse suction on tube to stop leakage
   Four tins of [company product]
   Five [Company brand] chocolate bars

Under 'Detailed plan':

   Finish items
   Go to Sydney
   Take computers, printer, and printer paper

Go to designated store in Sydney area
Check out caravan park near city
Go and scout store to be used as target
Go to different store and buy item
Back to caravan park
Fill in letter, details, print and disguise myself

Numerous other exhibits were located in the home, particularly in the bedroom, including various documents pertaining to the bank account and information about obtaining fake identifications. There were also syringes with needles, a Sydney tourist guide, rubber gloves, a list of the company's products on a pamphlet about boycotting it and an itemised list involving the preparation of a disguise.

Mills was then taken back to the St Kilda Road police complex where he was interviewed and formally charged with demanding money with menaces. Bail was refused. The following day he took part in an identification parade and the bank teller officially identified him. He was then extradited to Sydney to face the charges.

The whole episode, from the beginning of the investigation to Mills's arrest, had taken fourteen days. Not only was the food company extremely relieved, but two major food retailers expressed their appreciation and congratulated the police.

In November 1997 Mills pleaded guilty. He told the court that he had first contemplated this crime as the scenario for a novel he wished to write. He was sentenced to five years' gaol with a non-parole period of two years.

CHAPTER

12

Risk assessments

No two negotiations are the same.

In every case, the team needs to assess the risks involved to decide how the negotiation will be carried out. Each method has advantages and disadvantages. The deciding factors are the risks involved for the negotiator, any hostages and, of course, the general public. Taken into consideration are issues such as whether the subject has a weapon, if so, what type; whether the negotiator could become a target or a hostage; how the negotiator will liaise with other team members and how the question of the negotiator's personal safety can be addressed. Such issues need to be weighed up in deciding how advisable a face-to-face negotiation might be.

While I was working on the food extortion case in Sydney I was called out to a siege at Mays Hill, about twenty-five kilometres west of Sydney's CBD. Late one evening outside the local rugby club a man named Dave had assaulted his girlfriend, injuring her. During the assault Dave produced a knife and threatened to kill her.

Dave had left the area before the police arrived and his girlfriend told them he had probably gone home. She added that he was drunk and had knives, swords, a large bow and arrows and clubs at his home. Mindful of this, police went to Dave's home in Mays Hill. Dave was home but became very aggressive and the police were unable to arrest him. By now they had been told that he had been involved with firearms so they set up perimeters and called in the State Protection Group, the Tactical Unit and negotiators.

I was the primary negotiator, which meant I would be speaking with Dave. Because he was heavily armed, drunk and aggressive a face-to-face negotiation was considered too dangerous. We wanted to communicate with him as soon as possible but organising the negotiator truck would take time. Fortunately, an obliging neighbour was happy to let us use his home telephone. (There were no easy-access mobile phones in 1997.)

It was now after midnight. Once I knew the Tactical team were in place, I called Dave from the neighbour's house. The first telephone call is the most difficult and it is important to be very aware of the message you intend to give. I was not looking to resolve the situation, although that would have been nice, but to build up rapport with Dave and gather information about his state of mind and level of intoxication.

During our conversation it became apparent that Dave was very depressed and threatening to kill himself. This was of great concern because of the weapons he had, which he confirmed. He might have come charging out of the house with a gun in the hope police would shoot him, committing 'suicide by cop'.

We talked about his current situation, the events that had led to this, and the future. He wanted me to come into his home and sit down to talk with him, but I had to be honest with him, saying I couldn't because he was so heavily armed. I did tell him I would be happy to see him once he left the house safely.

After some hours he agreed to leave all his weapons inside and surrender to police. I agreed to meet him outside after police had searched him. It was very necessary to explain everything that would happen when he left the house so he was not surprised by anything. Besides, if in the future he did this again, he would know I had kept my word that he would not be harmed, and negotiators could remind him of this.

I told him to leave by the front door, unarmed, and to follow the instructions of the police dressed in black overalls. He knew I would be waiting near his front gate to meet him once Tactical police declared the situation safe. After this was made clear our telephone conversation ended.

I held my breath. The crucial moment had arrived, the time when you always hope you have read the situation correctly.

Dave came out of his front door and was met by the Tactical police. Thankfully no weapons were produced, and I could breathe again.

Dave was a massive bear of a man, nearly two metres tall and almost a metre wide, sporting a full beard, long hair and covered in tattoos. While he was being searched I walked to his front gate. Just as I had promised, I met with him and shook his hand. We both knew he was about to be taken to the police station and charged with the assault on his girlfriend, but I also knew it had taken him a lot of soul searching to find the courage to surrender instead of taking his own life.

A few months later while I was investigating a murder in the southern Sydney suburb of Kogarah I was called out to a siege situation that required a different approach. At a home unit in Carlton just south of Kogarah a thirty-seven-year-old man, Jack, had bashed his mother and was in his bathroom armed with a knife.

I had met Jack before. In October 1995 I had been called out as a negotiator to this same home unit where Jack was threatening to kill himself. He had been under the influence of drugs and alcohol, which did not help. On that occasion negotiations had failed and heavily armed Tactical police had arrested Jack, who was extracted kicking and screaming. I felt that this new situation would be difficult, not only because of Jack's nature but because of the circumstances surrounding his previous arrest.

On arrival at the block of units I saw that the Tactical police were organising their equipment. With the rest of the negotiation team I had a briefing from the general duty police, who had arrived first. They told us that there had been an argument between Jack and his mother, who also lived in the two-bedroom unit. Jack had hit his mother over the head with a blunt object, causing a large gash to her head which started bleeding profusely. He then kicked her in the back. She had been able to drag herself across the lounge room floor and across the foyer to alert a neighbour before losing consciousness.

The police found Jack sitting in the shower cubicle holding at thirty-centimetre carving knife and threatening to stab himself or the officers if they tried to arrest him. He had been drinking and appeared to be on some type of medication. A siege situation ensued and these police immediately called for the negotiators.

Our information was that Jack disliked women, was extremely racist and hated various police at Kogarah police station. Unfortunately, I was one of the negotiators, the secondary negotiator, John, was a sergeant from Kogarah whom Jack detested with a passion, and our fourth was an Italian.

It was decided that I would start negotiating with him face to face as soon as the Tactical police were in position. I put on a ballistic vest, as I would be very close to Jack. It was extremely dangerous, but there were not too many options and it would be helpful to see what Jack was doing.

The two-bedroom unit was small. There was a lounge room with a small hallway running off it to a bedroom. At the entrance to the bedroom the hallway turned right for approximately two metres ending at the entrance to a small toilet cubicle. Just before that was a doorway leading into the bathroom where Jack was.

I stood in the hallway outside the bathroom. There was very little room and the secondary negotiator, John, stationed himself in the toilet to my left, while the Tactical police positioned themselves opposite the bedroom doorway and around the corner to my right.

The bathroom door was open and I was directly opposite Jack. He was sitting in the shower cubicle holding the carving knife in one hand and a silver bladder from a wine cask in the other. There were opened packets of some type of medication on the floor of the shower cubicle, the glass door of which was shut.

It was less than one metre from the bathroom door to the shower cubicle. This was not going to be easy, I knew. Jack's state, under the influence of alcohol and whatever pills he was taking, would not help in negotiations. He also knew he would be arrested for the assault on his mother. Due to the danger of the situation, including the small, tight space he had squirmed into with the knife, it would be very difficult to arrest him without someone getting injured. The only option was to try and negotiate him out of the bathroom without the knife.

With this in mind I introduced myself to Jack. 'Hello, Jack. My name is Belinda Neil and I am a police negotiator. I would like to talk to you about an incident here earlier today. Firstly, are you okay?'

He replied, 'Just leave me alone. Why can't you all just leave me alone?'

I could tell from his voice, manner and eyes that he was heavily under the influence of drugs or alcohol. Fortunately, he didn't seem to recognise me from the previous incident. Now I had to negotiate with a drunk, never a good thing at the best of times.

During our conversation Jack informed me of his above-average intellect. He said he had just completed a master's degree in philosophy and studies in American criminology, amongst numerous other things. He had the superior air that can sometimes go hand in hand with high intelligence. I tried a number of different strategies, but nothing I said was getting through to him, and it was just making him more agitated.

At one point Jack asked, 'Can I come out and sit on the lounge and talk?' I told him yes, certainly, if he was prepared to leave the knife in the shower.

He said, 'I'm not leaving the knife here, those other cops told me it would be okay to bring it with me.'

I repeated that he must leave the knife behind him. He insisted that he had been told differently. I said, 'I will speak to those other police and see if there was a misunderstanding, but I would like you to promise me that you will not hurt yourself while I am gone.' He agreed.

That promise was important. Sometimes people in Jack's position feel that no one cares for them and they are on their own. Soliciting a promise from someone goes a long way in developing trust and strengthening the bond between negotiator and subject. It can show the person that the negotiator really does have their best interests at heart and it can be the first time a person feels that someone is really listening to them. It is important for the negotiator to convey that they care about the welfare of the person. The negotiator is not there to judge; rather, to try and ensure a peaceful resolution to a high-risk or crisis incident. Such a promise might also make the subject think about their own welfare rather than wanting to commit suicide. This is especially the case where there are hostages, the promise can help someone think about something else rather than the dire situation they are in.

The police denied telling Jack he could sit on the lounge with the knife and talk. This was a relief; we couldn't break promises but this was not one we could have kept.

After I had a short break to collect my thoughts, and a quick briefing with my team leader, I returned to the bathroom and told Jack what the police had said. He replied, 'Well they are liars, they promised me and they even gave it in writing.'

This was a surprise. 'Fair enough,' I said. 'Could you show me where they wrote it?'

Jack showed me a yellow sticky note with the promise written on it, signed by one of the police officers I had just spoken to.

That was certainly embarrassing for all involved and it meant another setback to negotiations. Needless to say I wasn't impressed with that particular police officer. Police credibility had now lessened, any attempt to build up trust and rapport was going to be more difficult. My job was now to try and rebuild what I had just lost.

Jack was rude, belligerent and aggressive. He kept repeating that he wanted police to kill him. 'Just shoot me like you shot Levi.' He was referring to an incident at Bondi a few months earlier when police had been confronted by Roni Levi, armed with a large kitchen knife, and had shot him dead.

The strategy I adopted was to talk to Jack about other areas of interest, to divert his mind from thoughts of suicide. This was difficult when I could see him drinking from the wine bladder and knew that he was getting drunker and drunker.

Every so often I felt a hand at my back, and John, my secondary negotiator, would pull me back slightly. I hadn't realised it but as I was talking to Jack I was moving closer to him. This is quite common, and the primary negotiator needs to have faith that the secondary negotiator is keeping an eye out for them. Jack couldn't see John, which was fortunate because he loathed him.

Jack grew more agitated and began tapping the carving knife blade against the door of the shower cubicle. He kept demanding cigarettes. We had been there for a couple of hours and had already supplied him with some. We were also becoming concerned at the medication he had taken and the amount of wine he had consumed. We decided that the next time he asked for a cigarette, we would not give him one until he had placed the knife outside the cubicle.

As primary negotiator I didn't make the decision how to respond but passed the request up the line to my team leader. He in turn passed it to the duty officer or commander, who made the decision based on my advice, as well as advice from the Tactical commander. This process was carried out for every request Jack made, even down to something as simple as asking for a cigarette. It was my job to negotiate that message across.

I had a very bad feeling that on this occasion the message was not going to be well received. Jack indeed became even more agitated, standing up and tapping the knife on the shower cubicle in my direction. He started making slicing movements across his neck with his thumb and threatening to stab and kill me.

'Get me a cigarette *now*.'

'Jack, put the knife outside the shower recess and I will get you a cigarette.'

'Get me a fucking cigarette or I will kill you.'

'Jack, I will not get a cigarette while you are holding the knife, so please put it outside the shower door.'

'Fuck you, I want a cigarette.'

'I'm happy to get you a cigarette, you just have to put the knife outside the shower.'

'I'm going to kill you.'

Jack continued to make threats towards me then he opened the door of the shower cubicle. Fortunately he remained where he stood and continued to wave the knife at me in a threatening manner yelling, 'I'm gonna stab you; get me a cigarette!'

At this stage he was just over a metre away, with nothing between him and myself but a large carving knife. The danger was reaching a critical point. In a calm voice I kept repeating that he should put the knife down.

I could see out of the corner of my right eye that the Tactical team was getting ready for a potential assault. I continued telling Jack to put down the knife. I knew I was in extreme danger, but I also knew I needed to try and stay in position to keep him talking and occupied until I was certain the Tactical team were ready. *Not long now, not long now, stay calm and just keep talking*, I told myself.

As Jack continued to yell and make stabbing motions like the killer in the shower scene of *Psycho*, everything zoned out for me except for my focus on him, the knife and staying calm. Then I felt Mick Coleman next to me on my right, and I knew they were ready. Mick was the pointman or lead Tactical officer, and as it was such a small hallway the others were lined up behind him and around the corner out of sight.

Suddenly Jack lunged at me from the shower cubicle with the carving knife in his right hand raised above his shoulder. I froze. I couldn't move. The knife was about thirty centimetres away from me when Mick pushed me out of the way at the same time John grabbed me and pulled me into the toilet recess. The Tactical boys rushed into the small bathroom and disarmed Jack, using tear gas, among other things. The can locked on and the gas, not having much room to spray out in the small bathroom, escaped into the hallway and toilet area. I felt its effects immediately, and my ears, nose and throat started to burn. I went straight outside into the fresh air.

Jack was arrested and taken away to Kogarah police station where he was charged with the assault on his mother, Mick and myself, among other charges.

Our negotiation team had a quick operational debrief then I drove the five minutes to Kogarah police station where I had been assisting detectives with Strike Force Apatin, a murder investigation. My Homicide work partner Angelo took one look at me when I arrived and said, 'Are you all right?' John had already arrived at the station and told my work partner that he had saved my life.

My first reaction was confusion. I felt annoyed that John had said that, but I think I was still in shock. Bloody hell, it *had* been close. Too close. I was still coming to terms with exactly what had happened. I couldn't understand why I hadn't moved when Jack lunged at me. Had I been so focussed on Jack and the knife that I hadn't had time to react? Had I just frozen as part of the 'fight or flight' response? I started to feel angry and frustrated as I couldn't answer this question and felt that this affected my professionalism. I also felt guilty that I could have endangered Mick as he had to push me out of the way to get at Jack.

A couple of days later I saw Mick when I went into the State Protection Group office to return the negotiation pager at the end of my on-call week. I asked if he was okay. He showed me his arms, bruised with scratches from the struggle in the bathroom. This did not help me, as I still felt confused by my actions.

Sometime later my negotiation team leader recommended that I receive a Commissioner's Commendation for Bravery 'arising from her outstanding courage and dedication that she displayed in the execution of her duty under such adverse and dangerous conditions'. A Commissioner's Citation was sought for the rest of the negotiation team and the Tactical team.

This preyed on my mind and I spoke to the commander about it. Yes, I had spoken to Jack for a good few hours in 'adverse and dangerous' circumstances where the threat level had remained high; yes, I had remained in position until I knew the Tactical team was ready. But I didn't feel it right or appropriate to accept any bravery award because I had frozen to the spot and still felt uncomfortable about this. I kept the original report so that it was never submitted; unfortunately this meant that the rest of the negotiation team and the Tactical team also missed out on recognition. My apologies particularly to Mick Coleman and John Hurley; thanks, guys.

This situation would give me flashbacks about how close I had come to being very seriously injured. It also showed me how much I had come to rely on the Tactical team and having them close by as a safety measure. Years later this too would play on my mind. when I returned to work at a Local Area Command.

CHAPTER

13

Psychopath

During August and September 1997 I continued working with Strike Force Apatin based at Kogarah. This had been established after the murder of Anthony Malouf, apparently the victim of a home invasion gone wrong, on 20 January that year at Brighton Le Sands. I spent the first two weeks assisting local Kogarah detectives, then Homicide support was scaled down and I returned to other investigations. Later that year there was a potential breakthrough in the Malouf case and Homicide assistance was needed. With my Homicide colleague Detective Senior Constable Angelo Memmolo (known as Ange), I returned to work at Kogarah.

I might add that at this time I was conducting inquiries into four other murders, including the shooting murder of Mark Rogers in 1988.

Mark Rogers had been the manager of the Rex Hotel in Kings Cross and was working on the day the hotel was robbed. He was shot in the back of the head with either a .45 calibre or 9mm firearm. The same firearm had also been used to kill a taxi driver at Ashfield in that same year. The Rogers murder had never been heard at inquest because there were still so many avenues of investigation to follow.

I worked on this case for three years on and off. During the investigation I interviewed a number of witnesses and suspects, and an informant was flown in from Queensland. The television program *Australia's Most Wanted* was also used to gather information. A listening device operation involving the main suspect was organised, but unfortunately there was not sufficient evidence for anyone to be charged. Finally after twelve years the inquest into the Mark Rogers murder was heard in the Coroner's Court, to the relief of Mark's long-suffering parents. The murder remains unsolved and the main suspect, who was serving a lengthy prison term for armed robbery, would have been released by now.

I felt I was drowning in paperwork. The staff officer at the Homicide Unit and I had a disagreement about my workload. He eventually agreed to take one of my murder cases, which I hadn't even had the chance to address, and forward it to another investigator. This respite was short-lived.

On Tuesday 30 September 1997 the crime manager at Kogarah police station asked Ange and me to look at a crime scene for him. A man had been found dead at his home in Allawah and local detectives were trying to decide whether it was a suicide or a suspicious death. Neighbours had reported hearing a noise like a single gunshot between 8pm and 9pm on the evening of the 27th, and a neighbour heard a car driving off shortly after the gunshot. The next morning a nine-year-old girl who lived nearby was walking past the man's house and saw him lying on the floor near the front door. She thought he was drunk and the blood on the wall was spilt red wine. She told her father what she'd seen but her father did not follow it up. Another neighbour became concerned after seeing a build-up of letters in his letterbox, and went to check on him on 30 September. Realising what had happened, he contacted police immediately.

When we got to the home we found the man lying on his back face upwards just inside the front door. He was wearing a dressing gown, socks and shoes. There was a large pool of blood near his head and what appeared to be a single gunshot wound to his jaw. A spent 9mm Norinco brand cartridge lay near his body.

I walked past his body along a hallway to the bathroom. There was blood on the walls and in the toilet bowl, along with unflushed faeces and a pair of underpants.

The detectives had searched his home and found documentation that identified him as Ronald Mills. We heard that Mills's wife had died on 26 August ten years earlier, that he was depressed about her death, and that he had made comments about life not being worth living.

Initially we thought he had shot himself in the bathroom, then dragged himself to the front door to get help and collapsed. The problem with that scenario was that there was no gun. We looked everywhere and located two older .22 calibre shotguns, but no 9mm gun. The two other firearms were later dismissed as possible weapons. It now looked very much like a suspicious death, but what was the motive?

Strike Force Coldwater led by Detective Senior Sergeant John Thompson of Kogarah was set up to investigate. As Ange and I were already working from Kogarah our Homicide office asked us to perform an oversight role, providing assistance and Homicide support where needed.

A post-mortem showed a partial contact gunshot wound to Ronald Mills's right jaw. The 9mm Norinco bullet had travelled down his neck, severing his jugular vein, and entered his left shoulder. The only lead we had was that Mills was listed as a witness in a boat insurance fraud case involving a man named Paul Offer. This fraud was listed for hearing on 13 October, eleven days away. In February Nagwa Gerges, the wife of another witness, had been shot non-fatally in the head with a crossbow at her front door. Paul Offer was starting to look very much like a potential suspect in both matters.

Investigators from the initial boat insurance fraud and from the Nagwa Gerges shooting were called in for briefings. At the same time, the strike force made inquiries into the current location of Paul Offer and the other witnesses in the fraud case, and applied for reverse call charge records from Ronald Mills's home telephone number.

We learned that Mark Gerges, the husband of Nagwa Gerges, owned a panel beating and spray painting business in the inner-city suburb of Rosebery. Paul Offer operated a tow truck in the southern Sydney suburbs and would drop off repair work to Gerges. Offer, an Irishman, was clearly a schemer who wanted to make money by any means possible, legal or otherwise. He had told Gerges and others stories about fighting for Britain in the Falklands and having been a member of the IRA. Many people were sceptical to say the least, though he appeared to have convinced himself that these stories were true.

Paul Offer and his family had visited Mark Gerges's home in St Ives. However, the two men had a falling out in October 1996 after Offer was charged with possession of stolen tools that he told police he had bought from Gerges. Gerges denied this and gave evidence on behalf of police. In November 1996 Crime Stoppers (a system that allows members of the public to report crime anonymously) received a tip from a man with an Irish accent that stolen property could be found at Gerges's panel-beating business. Police did find stolen property there: a piece of chassis rail, Victorian registration plates and vehicle compliance plates belonging to a stolen Isuzu motorhome that Paul Offer had rented and later reported stolen. Also found was a mobile telephone with the name 'Paul Offer' inscribed on it. Tit for tat, perhaps.

In retaliation a furious Gerges told police about a six-figure boat insurance fraud perpetuated by Offer. Police interviewed a number of people about this, including Ronald Mills, a marine electrician at Blakehurst Marina. Mills was able to identify the boat, a Mustang 3200, subject of the fraud. He could also confirm, as his marina was the Sydney agent for the Mustang 3200, that Paul Offer, whom he did not know, did not own any Mustang boats. Police also interviewed Offer's supposed accomplice, Armand Scerri, and in February 1997 both Scerri and Paul Offer were charged with fraud. We contacted Armand Scerri and re-interviewed him. It was obvious to us that he had been coerced by Offer.

Paul Offer was served with the police brief of evidence containing a witness list and the statements of all witnesses. There were statements from Mark Gerges, Ronald Mills and another man, Mark Chapman. These contained their business addresses and telephone numbers, and in the case of Mark Chapman, his home address and business address. (When serving a brief of evidence, addresses and telephone numbers of witnesses must always be deleted or blacked out.)

From the investigators of the Nagwa Gerges shooting we learned that shortly after midnight on Saturday 15 February

Mark Gerges and his wife Nagwa had both been at home at St Ives. Mark had been drinking with his brother and friends and had just bidden them goodnight. He was using the downstairs bathroom when Nagwa heard a knock at the front door. She opened the door and saw a tall man with green eyes, wearing a full balaclava and black gloves, pointing something at her. Without saying anything, he shot her at close range with a crossbow. The bolt struck her right between the eyes, pierced her skull and travelled through her brain. Mark, hearing her fall to the ground, ran to her aid. Without thinking, he pulled the bolt from her head with all the force he could muster, bending the shaft of the bolt in the process, then called the ambulance and police.

As a result of her husband's quick thinking, Nagwa survived the attack. However, she suffered severe head and brain injuries, including permanent semi-paralysis of her right side with moderately severe weaknesses in her right limbs, and problems with her vision and speech.

An anonymous tip told police they would 'find what you are looking for' at Mark Gerges's brother's panel-beating shop. Police did find four crossbow bolts, two similar to the one fired at Nagwa with red and black vanes, and two different-coloured ones. The bolts were found on top of a dusty spray booth but the bolts themselves were not dusty, suggesting they had been recently placed there.

The investigators interviewed Paul Offer about the shooting. He denied any knowledge, telling police that he, his de facto wife and three children had travelled by car from Sydney to the Gold Coast on 14 February, arriving at the Gold Coast the following morning in time to keep an appointment with a man from Nationwide Marine. For some reason this alibi was not followed up at the time. (Months later, Strike

Force Coldwater investigators spoke to the Nationwide Marine man who said there had never been any appointment with Offer.) Offer denied ever being in possession of a crossbow but told investigators he had seen a crossbow in Mark Gerges's garage.

The investigators narrowed their focus on the Gerges family and due to their marital problems Gerges became the prime suspect in his wife's shooting. However, there wasn't sufficient evidence to charge him.

Here was a classic case of tunnel vision. The investigators had not been open-minded to all possible suspects, nor had they followed up on all alibis. Even after we shared the information we had on the Mills murder and our view that Paul Offer was a suspect in both it and the Gerges shooting, they remained adamant that Mark Gerges was the prime suspect.

Given that we believed Offer had already killed or attempted to kill two witnesses in the boat insurance fraud court case it was crucial that we find him before he attacked other witnesses. Several Sydney addresses known to be connected with Offer were put under surveillance until we found out that Offer and his family had left Sydney in April 1997, five months earlier, and were believed to have headed north. The reverse call charge records on Ronald Mills's home telephone showed a call from Queensland on the evening of 29 September (two days after his death). This phone number was traced to a public phone box outside the Dress Circle Motor Village near the Gold Coast.

On Friday 10 October Detective Sergeant John Thompson, the officer in charge of Strike Force Coldwater, and another investigator from Kogarah were dispatched to the Gold Coast. At the Dress Circle Motor Village, the manager gave them a list of the names of everyone who had been there on

29 September 1997. Paul Offer was on the list. He was still living in the Motor Village with his de facto wife and children, in the Isuzu motorhome. The Queensland police were able to organise surveillance on him.

On 15 October 1997 they told us that the family appeared to be leaving town. It was time to act. The Homicide Unit gave Ange and me permission to drive the 800 kilometres to Brisbane to assist the Strike Force Coldwater investigators. It was more practical for us to take a car rather than fly; there were now four NSW investigators in Queensland and we didn't want to burden the Queensland police by using their resources. On arrival we met with the Queensland Armed Holdup Unit, who were helping us.

During the surveillance operation Sandra MacDonald, Paul Offer's de facto wife, agreed to come back to the police station with me to be interviewed. During the interview she provided alibis for Offer for the shooting of Nagwa Gerges and the murder of Ronald Mills, relying on diary entries she had made. Sandra told me that Offer had been with her at the Gold Coast on 15 February 1997, the day Nagwa Gerges was shot. On 27 September, the day Ronald Mills was killed, she claimed that Offer had been looking after their children while she was at work.

Paul Offer was also interviewed. He denied any involvement in the murder of Ronald Mills, stating that on Friday 26 September he had held a birthday party at the caravan park and recalled the caretaker fixing the barbecue they were to use for the party. On the night of the Mills murder, 27 September, he claimed he'd driven his wife to work at a hospital in Brisbane, where she was a nurse. Offer also denied possession of any firearms or ammunition, and denied knowing Ronald Mills.

When we followed up on Paul Offer's alibi at the Dress Circle Motor Village, a witness showed us a diary entry that noted Offer had driven his car to Sydney being absent from the motor village for two nights, returning on Sunday 28 September (the day after the shooting of Ronald Mills). Later, the investigation team located a hitchhiker who told us that Offer had picked him up on the way back from Sydney to Brisbane on 28 September. The manager of the Motor Village did remember fixing the barbecue for a birthday party, but it was for someone else's birthday two weeks before the date Offer had given. Video evidence showed Offer had been present at that birthday party on the 14 September, not 26 September as he had declared in his interview. We also found that Sandra MacDonald had taken taxis to and from work on 26 and 27 September, yet on 27 September a storage unit leased in her name at Kennards Hire in Kirrawee south of Sydney had been accessed twice by someone using the required key and code number.

Unfortunately, at the time of the interviews, we did not have enough evidence to charge either Offer or Sandra MacDonald.

We wanted Crime Scene to do a thorough forensic search of Offer's Ford Falcon car and Isuzu motorhome, to be video recorded. This could take days, even with numerous Forensics staff. Because it was late at night and not enough Forensics staff were available we decided to conduct this search the following day, Thursday 16 October. Offer and Sandra MacDonald were allowed to leave after we organised surveillance on them. They were travelling with children so we did not believe they could get far without our knowledge.

In the boot of the Falcon the following morning we found some very interesting items: a silencer capable of being threaded onto a 9mm pistol; a gun-cleaning kit that bank records showed had been bought on Offer's credit card; a sawn-off

shotgun; five crossbow bolts with red and black vanes similar
to those used in the shooting of Nagwa Gerges; a national
sports shooting brochure; Mark Chapman's business card and
a blank card with the Gerges' address written on it. There was
also a folder containing the brief of evidence for the forthcoming fraud case, including all the witness statements. A number
of sticky notes were attached to the statements, each one with
the name of the witness written on it. There was a cross under
Ronald Mills's name.

In the motorhome we located another disturbing exhibit.
This was a black zipped Commando brand bag that contained a Luger 9mm self-loading pistol in a brown holster
with a silencer fitting, seven rounds of Norinco brand 9mm
ammunition in the magazine fitted to the Luger, more 9mm
Norinco brand ammunition, a shoulder holster, a full balaclava with eye and mouth holes, black sunglasses and a black
bum bag. There was also a laser sight with mounting suitable
for attachment to a crossbow, black plastic zip ties (useful for
tying up prisoners), a piece of diamond-saw wire with swiv-
els and finger rings in each end, suitable for garrotting, and a
red-handled stainless steel diver's knife in a sheath. We called
this the assassin's kit.

We believed we had found the weapon used to kill
Ronald Mills, but to prove the murder charge we needed
to have the bullet, currently held in evidence in New South
Wales, analysed against the Luger 9mm pistol. One of the
Strike Force Coldwater investigators flew with the bullet to
Queensland ... and bingo. After test firing was carried out,
the murder weapon was confirmed.

Besides the assassin's kit we found a photograph of Mark
Gerges and his family, the home and business addresses of
Mark Gerges on a piece of paper, information about gun laws

in Queensland, two of Ronald Mills's Blakehurst Marina business cards, documentary proof that Offer had been in Sydney on 19 September and a Visa card cash advance slip for $8000 dated 25 September.

Paul Offer had claimed he did not know Ronald Mills but his mobile telephone records showed he had made many calls to Ronald Mills's workplace, and had called his home six days before the murder. He had made a further seven calls to the Sydney numbers of people named R Mills taken from the White Pages. Police contacted all these numbers, ensuring that their owners were safe and well. One person recalled that a man with an Irish accent asked for someone called Mills. In the motorhome, there was another interesting stash: 81 live rounds of 9mm Norinco ammunition wrapped in plastic, two boxes other containing 97 live rounds of 9mm Chinese Manufacture brand ammunition and a 9mm magazine loaded with seven live rounds of 9mm Norinco brand ammunition.

All this, of course, was very damning for Paul Offer. However, the surveillance police trailing Paul Offer had lost him; the family dog was found dead in a nearby park, butchered with a knife, and though we found Sandra MacDonald and the children with the hire car, Offer had fled. We needed to find him, and fast, before he left the country.

We knew he had been in contact with the owner of a large catamaran and were worried that Offer would try and find the owner, dispose of him/her, and take off with the boat to escape police. Perhaps this sounds a little melodramatic, but we were dealing with a man we strongly believed had killed one witness and tried to kill another over a boat fraud, and now he knew he was wanted for murder. We could not take unnecessary risks: Offer's potential to inflict major damage was too catastrophic.

From Brisbane I telephoned the owner of the catamaran, Mark, who told me he was moored in Sydney. He said he and his wife Katherine had met Paul Offer several times after Offer realised their boat was for sale and Offer had told them he wanted to buy the boat to sail back to Ireland. After some negotiation they eventually agreed on a sale price of nearly $500,000. Offer turned up to the boat with signed transfer forms but Mark had wanted to wait until settlement before handing the boat over. No money, no boat.

Several times Offer turned up and gave reasons for not having the money. Once he showed a photograph of hundreds of dollars in a briefcase (this photo was located in the motorhome). Mark and Katherine were becoming a little concerned, especially as Offer had asked them to go to the boat alone one night, promising to hand over the money. He had specifically asked them not to have their adult son with them. They also worried about the black bag he always carried but he told them it contained his dive suit, though they did not think the bag looked full enough. Chances are that bag was the assassin's kit.

Offer had contacted them a few days before, saying he was coming to Sydney and wanted to have dinner with them to settle the boat the following Monday – only three days away. Mark told Offer exactly where they were moored.

We now had a very serious situation. Offer was still missing, and he could be in Queensland or Sydney. What we did know was that he had a potential getaway plan that involved murdering Mark and Katherine. I did not mince words, telling Mark that Offer was wanted for murder and probably intended taking the boat to flee Australia. I also advised him, though not in these words, that he needed to up-anchor immediately and get the hell out of there, to find a suitable mooring then get off the boat and stay at a motel. I then rang the Sydney Water Police and advised them of the situation. They were fantastic and contacted Mark straight away. While I was satisfied that for the time being Mark and Katherine were safe, I would not feel fully at ease until Offer was located or I received confirmation that this couple were off their boat and in a discreet motel.

The following day surveillance police located Offer heading towards Brisbane airport. He was arrested for the murder of Ronald Mills and extradited to Sydney. I called Mark to let him and Katherine know that Paul Offer had been arrested. They could finally relax, as did I, knowing they were safe. It was time for us to return to Sydney and continue gathering evidence against Offer.

A few days later a Sydney man named Eric, said he was a friend of Offer's who had worked with him in the security industry many years before, contacted us saying he had read the newspaper reports of Offer's arrest. Eric told us that when they went drinking he and his friends used to laugh at Offer's stories of being an IRA hitman. As a joke Eric had told him that he was a hitman himself. Eric wanted to talk to us.

He told us that in early September 1997, after five or six years of no contact, Offer rang telling Eric he was in trouble and needed people 'taken care of'. Eric, who had never taken Offer seriously, thought he would just go along with the joke. Offer had mailed to him the names and addresses of three men, and, though Eric had thrown the list away, he recalled an Allawah address (Ronald Mills) and a Drummoyne address (Mark Chapman). Eric also remembered Offer saying that the men were witnesses in a boat fraud.

After this Offer called a number of times, offering him $10,000 for killing the three people on the list: Mills, Gerges and Chapman. Eric, who had no intention of doing anything of the kind, grew tired of Offer's calls and began to make excuses as to why he hadn't killed anyone. In mid September he met Offer, who told him again that he was in trouble and needed Eric's help. On 8 October – five days before the boat fraud case was due to start – he met Offer again, and Offer said, 'I've got one that I need fixed up desperately by the weekend.' He gave Eric the name and address of Mark Gerges.

As Eric was getting into Offer's car he saw a pistol in a brown holster on the back seat. Eric took the pistol out of the holster, recognising it as a 9mm Luger. Offer told him the gun was his and put it on the floor of the car, covering it with a coat.

Before Eric came to see the police, Paul Offer had telephoned him asking Eric to visit him in gaol and making veiled threat that Eric's fingerprints were on the gun used to kill Ronald Mills. Eric agreed to assist police and wear a listening device whenever he visited Offer.

Eric had four meetings with Paul Offer at Silverwater gaol and was wired up each time. We followed Eric to Silverwater and met him straight afterwards. Offer confirmed that he had asked Eric to kill three people, as well as the amount he was to pay. We confirmed that $8,000 had been withdrawn from Offer's Visa account two days before Ronald Mills's murder. The money was repaid on 29 September.

Offer further incriminated himself during conversations with Eric, saying, 'You kept putting me off so I took it into my own hands.'

He admitted to Eric that the police had found his weapons: 'They've got me, they've got me with the fucking guns, they've got me with the shotty in the car.'

He told Eric that he and Sandra MacDonald were creating a false alibi to show that Offer was in Brisbane at the time of Mills's murder and that he still needed, 'at least two fuckers to stitch Mark [Gerges] up'. He also asked Eric to help Sandra MacDonald get rid of a package that was in storage in Sydney, telling Eric this package contained the objects used to shoot Nagwa Gerges. 'The object that's in the storage right, was used on his missus ... she came to the door and she stepped in the way.'

On the morning of 31 October we followed Eric and Sandra MacDonald to Kennards in Kirrawee where the package was stored. Sandra retrieved a box which she gave to Eric to 'get rid of'. She told Eric that Offer had shot Nagwa Gerges by mistake. Sure enough the package contained a crossbow, seven bolts with metallic shafts and red and black vanes – the same type used to shoot Nagwa Gerges – and a black balaclava.

Because Eric was playing such a dangerous role, we decided to bring in an undercover police officer. Eric introduced this officer to Paul Offer as someone who could help him, and the officer had a number of conversations with Offer and Sandra MacDonald about false alibis for Offer. Sandra Mac-Donald spoke with a number of people to arrange false alibis for Offer for the night of Ronald Mills's shooting, even using a private investigator. She admitted to the undercover police officer that she knew Offer was in Sydney on the night that Ronald Mills was shot, and said Offer had told her he shot Nagwa Gerges and asked her to get rid of the crossbow. This contradicted what she said to me when I interviewed her in Queensland.

On 18 December I went to the home where Sandra Mac-Donald was staying and told her she was under arrest. She did not comment, only speaking to organise a carer for her children. She was charged with being an accessory after the fact to the shooting of Nagwa Gerges, and intention to pervert the course of justice because of the false alibis she had organised. She pleaded guilty at the Supreme Court and was sentenced to two years' gaol. She subsequently lost her children and refused all contact with Paul Offer.

Offer was still trying relentlessly to find a way out of the mess he was in. When he found out about the assistance Eric had given police, he made over twenty false allegations implicating Eric in the shooting of Nagwa Gerges and Ronald Mills and in other murders, as well as lying about Mark Gerges, Ronald Mills and the detective sergeant in charge of the investigation. He even tried to involve other prisoners in setting up Eric, telling Police Internal Affairs that all the investigators were dealing in drugs, finding someone to burn down the Gerges family home, and even putting out a contract worth $20,000 to kill Eric and the police investigators.

A great deal of incriminating evidence was found in his cell, including statutory declarations allegedly signed by Eric (his signature was later found to have been traced) admitting guilt for the murder and attempted murder. He also gave written descriptions of Eric and Mark Gerges for the benefit of whoever he was asking to do them harm. As a result he was charged with an additional three counts of soliciting to murder.

This case had started out as a relatively small insurance fraud and had developed into murder, attempted murder, soliciting to murder and taking contracts out on witnesses and police. The lengths to which Paul Offer went in his scheming astounded us. He may yet find a prisoner who believes his lies and will take him up on one of the contracts.

Offer had vehemently denied the charges against him. However, on the first day of his trial at the NSW Supreme Court he pleaded guilty to everything. On 29 June 2000 he was sentenced to thirty-four years in prison, with the earliest parole date 16 October 2022.

Offer's reign of terror had ended but his path of devastation remained. Families had lost a loved one. Nagwa Gerges never fully recovered from her physical injuries and she still suffers from major depression, insomnia, alternating mood swings and impairment to concentration. Others realised how close they had come to meeting their fate – Mark Chapman, the other witness Offer had earmarked for death, and Mark and Katherine, the owner of the boat and his wife, who had a lucky escape.

This case also highlights the potential danger to police officers, as we place ourselves at risk going to work every day. A police video made when Offer was first arrested driving the motorhome shows him talking to detectives while moving gradually towards the unlocked side compartment in which the assassin's kit, including the loaded Luger pistol, was later found. If given the chance would Offer have grabbed the pistol and shot his way out? I am sure of it: he was a man willing to do anything to achieve his goals. Fortunately he did not get the chance.

It is important to ensure our personal safety and the safety of our families, especially when dealing with some of the state's most dangerous criminals. The detective sergeant in charge of the investigation never returned to work after being named in the contract to kill him. This had gone beyond work – it was now personal and his family had been in danger. For him it was one dangerous job too many.

CHAPTER

14

Motherhood

A few months before the murder of Ronald Mills, Rob and I had decided it was time to start a family. Rob had wanted children as soon as we were married, but I'd wanted to achieve some milestones in my career first. Now I wondered about the impact of becoming a mother. My work with Homicide involved lots of time away from home working long hours or being called to investigations anywhere in New South Wales. On top of that, I had my negotiator work, although that was only part-time.

After being accepted into the Homicide Unit and becoming accredited as a counter-terrorist negotiator, I felt I had achieved two major goals. I was now twenty-nine years old and it was time to think about having children. I knew once I fell pregnant the kinds of work I did would need to be

reconsidered. For example, I would no longer be interviewing
suspects in case my protruding belly became a target.

Rob was on shift and working plenty of overtime at the
State Protection Group, Tactical Operations Unit, and I was
at the Homicide Unit, with trips away around the country.
We were rarely at home at the same time. After the initial
trip to Queensland in pursuit of Paul Offer we finally had
a weekend together which, very fortunately, resulted in my
becoming pregnant. We decided not to inform anyone until
I was at least twelve weeks along in case of miscarriage. I
rarely suffered from morning sickness and when I did found
that eating a few dry crackers helped.

While I was still putting together the brief of evidence
regarding Paul Offer and Sandra MacDonald (she had not
yet been charged), a good friend of mine, BP (see Chapter 2) asked whether I would be involved in an undercover
job involving a major cocaine-importing ring based in Canberra. I had worked with BP at the Undercover Unit back
in 1989, and he was now one of the supervisors. The job
would only require me to have a few meetings with the main
drug importer and the informant, then fly to Tahiti with
them and bring back cocaine. The informant, a stripper and
exotic dancer, had been asked by the drug importer to be
a mule and to find a friend to bring along for the free trip
to Tahiti. That friend would now be me and I was bringing
along my 'boyfriend'. The whole job should be over within
two weeks.

Rob and I decided it would be okay, as I was only five
weeks pregnant. My supervisors at the Homicide Unit had
to agree as well, and after some negotiation they agreed on
the grounds that the job would be short. So, at the end of
November, after false passports and driver's licence had been

organised, I set off to Canberra with another full-time under-cover operative – my 'boyfriend'– and BP.

As well as meeting with the Australian Federal Police offi-cers who were running the job, I needed to meet the informant so we could work out our cover story. After consultation with my undercover supervisor we decided not to say I had worked with her as an exotic dancer in case the drug importer wanted a performance to authenticate my profession. We decided I would be a long-standing friend of hers, not a stripper.

Unfortunately the informant had already told the drug dealer I was a stripper. If he wanted me to demonstrate, I was going to have to do some pretty fast talking. Not being par-ticularly flexible, about the only convincing equipment I had were full breasts, courtesy of the first trimester of pregnancy, and long legs.

I met the informant, a petite woman with a great body, and we worked out our cover story. Then with her and my alleged boyfriend I went off to meet the drug importer in suburban Canberra. I was a bit taken aback to discover that he was a big Islander lad, more than 1.8 metres tall and wide with it. Fortunately he accepted what we told him. We met twice more over the next two weeks and he gave various excuses why the flights to Tahiti hadn't been booked. I was starting to wonder whether the job would come off at all but had little time to think about it, being busy with Homicide investigations.

By Christmas nothing more had happened so I took a couple of weeks' leave. On return to work I went to Can-berra for further meetings with the importer. He introduced a friend who would be accompanying us. Wow. This man was another Islander about two metres tall and one and a half metres wide, and all of that was muscle, not an ounce of fat. I remember saying to the drug importer, 'I'm glad he's on our side.' The plan had now changed; we were now to travel to Houston, Texas to pick up the drugs.

By the end of January I spoke to BP and told him I was pregnant. I knew the trip would have to take place soon or I would be showing a nice pregnant belly, not exactly what was required in this situation. Then things went quiet with the importer and next we knew a shipload of drugs, which he was involved in, had been seized in Queensland. The job was off, the trip was off, and the importer was arrested for conspiracy to import drugs as a result of our investigation.

The next time I saw him was when I had to give evidence at his initial trial in Canberra Supreme Court. I was heavily pregnant so I was on tenterhooks at the thought of seeing him. This area was open to the public. I was concerned, not only that he would see me but that if he was angry enough to rush at me there would be no stopping him because he was so big.

I was also afraid he might organise for someone to dissuade me in a very violent way from giving evidence against him; I now had an unborn baby to protect. At least I walked in with BP and the Crown prosecutor so I was not on my own.

On this occasion the importer sacked his defence so the trial was put off until later in the year and I could leave Canberra immediately. When the trial was finally held at the Supreme Court in Canberra, he was convicted and sentenced to ten years' gaol for conspiring to import cocaine.

In January 1998 I told the commander of the Homicide Unit I was pregnant and duly signed an alternative duties form, which meant I was not to interview any potential offenders. I could now catch up on finalising briefs of evidence and other paperwork connected to my investigations. Ange and I went to Queensland to gather statements for the Paul Offer and

Sandra MacDonald briefs; I travelled to Goulburn to role-play on the negotiators' course and a drug trial involving 496 ecstasy tablets came up. On that one I got a conviction. Score one for the good guys.

I was due to give birth in July so I took some time off to try and relax beforehand. Nobody tells you about sleeplessness before the baby is born, or that you are up a few times at night going to the toilet. Perfect preparation for night-time feeds, though.

My baby was due on 19 July and my obstetrician decided to induce him due to his size. Approximately sixteen hours later Jake was coaxed out with forceps.

The obstetrician placed my beautiful son on my chest. It was an amazing moment; this tiny little creature was my son. His little face was screwed up and screaming, perhaps from a headache as a result of the forceps. All my tiredness and pain from the birth dissolved when I looked at him and I was left with an overwhelming feeling of protectiveness for him.

Then he was taken from me! The obstetrician told me he was going to send Jake for a check-up in the special care nursery because of breathing difficulties. As the midwife took Jake out of the room I had an overpowering feeling that I might never see him again.

I felt trapped, I couldn't get off the bed so I looked at Rob and said, 'Follow that baby.'

Rob hesitated and said he wanted to stay with me. I looked straight at him and repeated urgently: 'Follow that baby.' I think Rob must have picked up on my feelings as he left immediately. I was so concerned that Jake might be kidnapped that until I knew all the proper identification procedures had taken place and I was satisfied he was not in any danger, I didn't want him out of our sight.

My work experiences and associated fears were infiltrating my most precious moments, moments that should have been filled with happiness and joy. The panic and anxiety I was feeling – the fear that my baby might have been stolen from me – might possibly be considered normal for first-time mothers. However, the intensity and severity of these feelings shocked me. I didn't realise at the time that I needed help; these panic states, this fear being completely out of character for me, can most likely be interpreted as the early signs of hyperarousal, the initial stages of post-traumatic stress disorder.

I spent the next four nights with Jake next to my bed; I was determined not to let him out of my sight. By the fifth night the nurse came to take him to the respite nursery as I was not getting any sleep, so fearful was I that someone would come in and take him. I eventually gave in and slept until the nurse came and woke me to feed him. I finally relaxed when I got to take him home.

It was staggering how protective I felt about this little being in my life. This almost overtook all other feelings and it diminished the resources I had. I spent so much time worrying about the awful things that might happen to him that I had little time for the pleasure of watching him grow, watching him smile; getting excited when he smiled after five or six weeks and knowing it was because he was pleased to see me and not because of wind pain; watching the delight he took in exploring his surroundings, feeling and touching things. I had lost the ability to enjoy these moments.

I was now thirty years old. I had no idea about motherhood, having always been a career-minded girl, and definitely no maternal instincts, but I did read a lot of books. The five months I spent full time with my son was an amazing experience, although I don't profess for a minute to say it was easy.

I knew I would find it very hard to leave him and go back to work.

We had agreed that Rob would take six months off from the State Protection Group to look after Jake while I returned to work. He was hyped up, not sleeping properly and coming home irritable, often flaring up over the slightest things. I had always been a very patient person but my patience levels were sorely tested now and this created tension in our marriage, especially as I was trying to look after Jake too. The time off would be a good chance for Rob to have some time out and to think about the possibility of transferring out of the State Protection Group, as well as spending bonding time with our son. At this time, we didn't know that Rob, too, was displaying all the symptoms of post-traumatic stress disorder, and we didn't even consider counselling for him.

I returned to work in January 1999. I am going to say this to all the mothers out there — going back to work was like going on a holiday. At work I was not checking feeding or sleeping times or worrying about what Jake was doing. And while I had loved every minute of my very special bonding time with Jake I had never really relaxed. I think stay-at-home mothers are amazing, but that is a lifestyle choice for all concerned and not everybody has that opportunity.

The first night I came home from work I was feeling great, I felt intellectually stimulated. However, as soon as my car pulled into the drive, Rob flew out of the front door with his dog, Conan, a Jack Russell, in tow. His face was taut and angry.

Before I could say anything he said, 'I'm taking the dog for a walk,' and then he was gone.

I had no idea what had happened. I went into the house; Jake was sleeping and there was no dinner prepared. After an hour Rob returned, visibly cooled off, but he offered no explanation as to his immediate departure.

The next day I went to work stressed wondering what would I find when I got home. Would we have to reconsider our leave and look at other options? That evening I returned home tense and anxious. I opened the front door and the smell hit me: a baked dinner. I relaxed; all was well.

After my return to full time work in January 1999 I decided to leave the Homicide and Serial Violent Crime Agency (as the Homicide Unit was now called). I didn't feel I would be able to cope with an investigation into the death of a baby or child, and being asked to go anywhere in the state at short notice could also present a problem. A number of detective sergeant positions were being advertised throughout the state so I decided to apply for one of those close to home, and if I was unsuccessful I would apply for a lateral transfer instead.

Although the positions I sought were investigative, they were not specific to Homicide investigation but involved other kinds of crime, including armed robbery, sexual assault, fraud, and drug investigation for example. I was tired of being totally immersed in violence and death and looked forward to a change.

In September 1999 I successfully applied for the position of investigations manager, at detective sergeant level, at Kogarah Local Area Command. However, I would not be released from my current job until the following January.

While I had decided to leave Homicide, I couldn't bear to give up my negotiator's role as well. I found the work incredibly interesting, and particularly enjoyed the professionalism and working within a strong cohesive team. I also felt that I could make a difference. This did put me under extra pressure now Jake was born, but as a police officer this was work truly close to my heart. There was an amazing bond between negotiators. It didn't matter that the pager went off at 2am after little sleep, because I wanted to get out of bed and go to the job whatever it entailed. Having a partner who understood the work I was doing definitely helped.

For the first six months when I went back to work full time this was relatively uncomplicated as Rob was on leave. However, when he went back to work we had to do some quick thinking when I was on call as negotiator. Rob was often late for work as he had to drop Jake off at the child-care centre because I had been called out and had not arrived home in time. It was very helpful that my mother lived close by (she and Dad had separated some years before and he was now living and working in Fiji). She provided help whenever she could.

On the morning of 1 June 1999 various teams of police were searching premises throughout Sydney because of a major Kings Cross drug syndicate. The head of the syndicate was Michael Kanaan, currently on bail after being involved in a shootout with police at the White City tennis complex near Paddington in December of the previous year. One police officer had been shot and Kanaan himself was now confined to a wheelchair. Because he was considered dangerous and in possession of firearms, a team of police negotiators was involved when Kanaan's home in Bruce Avenue Belfield was to be searched.

If police are carrying out a normal search with a warrant, they will knock on the front door. For a high-risk search warrant the usual procedure is for Tactical police to surround the home and for negotiators to speak with the occupants on the phone or by some other means to ensure that the occupants leave the house safely. There is always the chance that they will refuse to come out and a siege will ensue. On this occasion that is exactly what happened. Kanaan refused to come out.

About 10pm, as I was getting ready for bed, the commander Graeme Abel rang me. The siege at Belfield was well and truly under way and did not look like being resolved in the next few hours. He needed to put together a second team of negotiators to relieve the initial team who had been working for nearly fourteen hours, and I agreed to lead that second team.

On arrival I saw the Tactical teams and the negotiators' truck. The Tactical teams were heavily armed; Kanaan was a suspected killer and the boys were not going to pull any punches should negotiations fail. In the negotiators' truck was Radar, leader of the first team, who looked exhausted. In the truck I saw numerous empty coffee cups and cartons of stale cold leftover McDonald's, and noticed the faint smell of body odour. It had been a long day.

Radar and Graham briefed me and I learned more about Michael Kanaan. He was a career criminal, a hardened drug dealer and gang leader. He was suspected of the shooting deaths of two men as well as murdering his own former gang leader Danny Karam. Then there was the shootout with police at White City. This later earned him fair coverage in the television series *Underbelly 3*.

When the rest of my team arrived we discussed strategies with the shortly-to-be-relieved morning team. Our main aim was to try and resolve the negotiation peacefully and our initial step was simply to use a new negotiator to see if there was more chance of rapport. Kanaaan had smashed the landline phone in his house, so we had to communicate from the negotiator's truck via a special telephone that had been thrown into the house, one that was much hardier and better able to sustain ill treatment.

Over the next twelve hours Kanaan constantly abused Glenn, my primary negotiator. It was amazing how Glenn kept his cool, but this is one of the skills of a good police negotiator. I had constant briefings with the Tactical team leader and also the operation commander to discuss strategies after most of these telephone calls. Exchanging information with the Tactical commander was important; the Tactical teams might see or hear things we couldn't, and we could also pass on information that might be helpful in carrying out various action plans.

These fall into two main categories. An Emergency Action plan (EA plan) is devised within thirty minutes of arrival if an emergency situation becomes life-threatening. For example, if the suspect starts killing hostages or threatening to detonate a bomb, the EA Tactical team may be deployed immediately into the stronghold. A Deliberate Option (DO) is a more detailed plan that may use additional resources as the incident continues. It is established within two hours of arrival and is continually updated and revised as more resources and intelligence become available. The DO may include a more detailed plan for breaching a stronghold and require more Tactical team members and outside agencies than the EA.

The media were breathing down our necks just waiting for a gunfight between Kanaan and Tactical police. We were not looking for a quick fix as that was too dangerous and more likely to end in a shootout. However the following morning, an assistant commissioner arrived with her entourage. They asked me why negotiators were not just ordering Michael Kanaan and his family out of their home and why police were not storming the place.

I was a little surprised by the question and wondered whether the overtime budget had become such an issue that human life came second to the desire to fast-track an arrest. I had been awake since six the previous morning, and perhaps I was a little terse as I reminded the assistant commissioner and entourage that the NSW police guidelines specified 'contain and negotiate' as the first response. I pointed out that storming the house could lead to deaths and the possibility of very damaging publicity for the police, and said that at least everybody was alive and unhurt. Well, nearly everybody: the assistant commissioner's ego was perhaps bruised. I was lucky not to be transferred somewhere else.

By 10.30am the following morning Radar and the initial team were called back to the siege to take over from us, as we had been operating for over twelve hours, some of us working through from the previous day. We were well and truly exhausted and after briefing the oncoming team and debriefing our own we left the area, knowing full well we might be back later that day if the siege continued.

Fortunately it ended later that afternoon with nobody hurt. Michael Kanaan was arrested peacefully and is currently serving three life sentences for murder.

Which brother?

In November 1999 I felt I had been coping reasonably well with full-time Homicide investigation but I was still counting the days before I could transfer to Kogarah Local Area Command. However, a case came along that changed my perception of the world. At that stage, though I did not know it, my mind was filling with all the traumatic memories of horrific investigations. At some stage I would overload. This case saw the beginning of that overload.

On Wednesday 3 November I started a normal 8am to 4.30pm shift at the Homicide Unit. I had just completed an on-call negotiator week, dropped off the pager that morning and was filling out job sheets for situations that included a man dousing himself with petrol before mutilating himself and a man wanting to jump off a rooftop. Both men had been taken for psychiatric assessments. That night I went to bed early and was probably asleep by 9.30pm. At 11.30pm my lovely rest was disturbed by a phone call from Detective Sergeant Russell Oxford, my Homicide team leader. A woman had been found murdered in her home at Berala and I was to meet him at her address.

When I met Russell, he looked at me and said, 'How can you be smiling after getting out of bed at this hour?' By then I was used to getting out of bed at all hours to go to Jake, so when I was called out I needed no time to become fully alert. An adrenalin surge kicked in very quickly even if I had only been asleep for a few hours.

Investigators from Flemington Local Area Command (LAC) told us that thirty-year-old Donna Wheeler had been brutally bashed and stabbed in her home. Her body had been found by her ex-husband and, tragically, by her twelve-year-old son, both of whom had been taken to Flemington police station to make statements. When Donna's son was asked what he saw when he went into the room, he said, 'My mother was laying in the lounge room in the corner with all blood up against the wall, and no pants on. Basically Dad got me out of there straight away.' I felt overwhelming pity for this poor child.

It was decided that Nigel (another Homicide investigator) and I would go back to Flemington to assist the young investigators who were taking statements from Donna Wheeler's son and ex-husband while Russell Oxford remained at the crime scene. Incredibly, the commander would not allow the detective sergeant at Flemington LAC to attend the crime scene due to overtime restrictions. Detective Sergeant Jenkins, who would start at 8.30 the next morning, would be put in charge of the homicide investigation nearly twelve hours after it began. The most important information in a homicide is usually obtained in the first forty-eight hours, often involving an enormous amount of detail. Trying to play catch-up twelve hours later would be very difficult.

Nigel and I discovered that Donna had taken out an apprehended violence order (AVO) against her ex-boyfriend, Keith Bond. He had been physically violent towards her during the relationship and had not been happy when she ended it. In fact, Keith appeared to be obsessed by Donna. Even with the AVO in place, it was believed he slashed the tyres on her car. Bond lived in Amy Street, Regents Park, with his brother Colin and another man, Peter, only a short distance from Donna's home at Berala. He became our number-one suspect.

Armed with this information we went to Keith Bond's home address in Regent's Park. It was 7.30am on Thursday 4 November. We had been working all night but now wasn't the time to stop. No one answered the door and it appeared no one was home. After a quick conversation with neighbours we decided to come back later. At that point we were going to view the crime scene at 9 Kingsland Road.

I have absolutely no independent recollection of the crime scene, as shocking as it was; by this stage I had internalised as much horror as I could handle. I have taken the following description from diaries, statements and photographs.

The fibro home was small with a carport in which was parked a red Mitsubishi Lancer. This was Donna's car. The front door of the house led to a small hallway with a bedroom on the right and the lounge room on the left. At the entrance to the lounge room I saw the brutally murdered body of Donna Wheeler.

She was lying on her back with her head towards a corner of the room but it was her face that drew my attention. It was covered in blood and swollen and bruised as if she had been hit by a hard object. Next to her head were a pillow and plastic bag, both covered in blood. A blood spray pattern was on the wall above her head. I felt numb: it was such a shocking sight and I knew her young son had seen his mother like this.

Her body was naked from the waist down apart from a black sock on her right foot, and her legs were spreadeagled. I felt as I had at the Paula Brown and Kim Meredith crime scenes: why couldn't her killer have covered her up? Why rob her of her dignity in death? The other sock lay near her black underpants and slacks on the carpet near her feet. Her hands were covered in blood. Her maroon top was also covered in blood and there were three holes or cuts in the top left side, which we later discovered hid stab wounds to her chest. There was also one stab wound and smears of blood on her abdomen.

In another corner of the room lay a small bloodied knife with a thirteen-centimetre blade. It was slightly bent, perhaps from hitting bone. From the positioning of her body, the knife and various items strewn around the room, it was obvious a violent struggle had taken place.

On the coffee table were three partly eaten Chinese take-away meals, two ceramic eating bowls and a bottle of Tooheys beer. Two spoons and forks were on the floor and another bottle of beer and a can of UDL were at the base. Who did Donna have her last meal with? And what or who had interrupted dinner for two that evening? There was no sign of forced entry to the home.

After reviewing the crime scene we returned to Amy Street Regents Park. This time Keith Bond's brother Colin was at home, and he let us in. Colin told us that Keith was not at home but would be at work. The other occupant of the house, Peter, was also absent. Russell asked Colin when he had last seen Donna.

Colin replied, 'Tuesday night I met her at the pub and then we had some Chinese at her place.'

'What time did you leave there?'

'About 7.30, or eight she got a phone call and she had to leave to meet someone at Ashfield.'

Russell also asked Colin about the relationship with Donna and his brother Keith.

Colin replied, 'There were heaps of blues.'

One of the investigators noticed what appeared to be a spot and smear of blood on the floor in the lounge room. At that point Russell had a short interview with Colin, recorded on tape. Whilst we had believed Keith was our main suspect and Colin even inferred this, Colin himself was not beyond scrutiny. He had known Donna and appeared to be one of the last people to see her alive. The fact that he admitted having eaten a Chinese meal with her was very significant. I also noticed that Colin's right hand seemed quite swollen. So now we had two very good suspects for the murder.

Keith had been in a tempestuous relationship with Donna, which had ended some weeks prior to her death. He had a history of violence towards her. Then we had Colin, who had been seen in Donna's company for the past couple of weeks. We learned that he had been released from gaol on parole some months earlier after serving ten years for bashing another woman in the face and leaving her for dead, naked from the waist down.

When Colin had been interviewed about the attack on this woman he said, 'With a few beers under my belt, I got the shits and hit her.' This had not even come close to what took place. The man who found this woman said she was 'gurgling', and that her face had been so badly beaten it appeared 'just pulped.' She had died sixteen days later. This crime scene also indicated that the woman might have rejected his sexual advances. However, Colin was adamant Donna that had taken a call and left to go and meet someone. We had to work out which brother had been responsible for her death – or whether the murderer had been the person Donna had left to meet at Ashfield.

Colin agreed to accompany detectives to Flemington police station to be interviewed further, and we made numerous phone calls to try and track down Keith and Peter, the other occupant of the home. Keith had a new girlfriend, Debbie, so we were trying to contact her as well. We also needed to organise a search warrant for the house where the Bond brothers lived.

Later that day Keith Bond presented himself at Flemington police station. It was decided that Russell would interview Colin Bond with a detective from Flemington and Detective Sergeant Glen Jenkins, the newly appointed officer in charge of the investigation, would interview Keith Bond with me. I felt for Glen, who was trying to catch up on the wealth of information that was flowing in at that time. He asked me to conduct the interview as he felt that he was 'behind the eight ball'.

I activated the video and tapes and started the two-hour interview with Keith. He said that at the time of the murder he had been with his current girlfriend, Debbie, whom he had met shortly after breaking up with Donna.

'Can you tell me why you broke up?' I asked.

'It was just the arguments that we were having and that, 'cause I went up, I ended up going on assault charge on her and we just broke up ...'

On the afternoon of Tuesday 2 November, Melbourne Cup Day, Keith said he and Debbie had been at the Regents Park

Bowling Club. About 7pm or just after, Keith left and went to the Regents Park Hotel leaving Debbie to play bingo. Donna and Colin had been at the hotel when he arrived. They left and Colin returned, and Donna came back just before nine. (This was later found to be consistent with telephone calls to Donna's phone but inconsistent with Colin's story.) Keith then left and went back to the bowling club to meet Debbie. They stayed there together until about ten, then a friend gave them a lift to Keith's home in Amy Street, where they went to bed.

'Did you see Colin again that night?'

'No I didn't, I heard him come in later on that night.'

'Can you tell me what time that was?'

'Not offhand, no. But I heard the front door go. Then I was awakened about twenty past twelve with the washing machine going.'

'Who was doing the washing?'

'I think it was Colin.'

'Why?'

'Well, Pete was in bed, I walked past his door and he was in bed.'

'How long had the washing machine been going?'

'Probably only a few minutes, 'cause I looked at the clock and it woke Debbie as well.' He added that he got up and turned the machine off, and he and his brother argued about it.

In a second interview some days later Keith said he had looked inside the washing machine and seen clothes as well as Colin's sandshoes.

Colin Bond admitted he had been with Donna that evening. They took some Chinese takeaway to her house with two bottles of Toohey's beer for him and a can of vodka and orange for her. They ate most of the meal but about 8.30pm Donna received a phone call and said she was going to Ashfield.

This timing was important. We were trying to ascertain whether Colin had been the last person to see Donna alive. We would need to confirm whether or not Donna had been telephoned, if so, at what time, and who the caller was. Colin said Donna dropped him home and that was the last time he saw her. He also said Keith and his girlfriend were at home in bed as he had heard them talking, confirming Keith's alibi. Later that night for no apparent reason Colin had decided to wash his clothes. He told police he had felt sorry for Donna because of the way Keith had treated her during and after their relationship. He even said he had 'belted' Keith one night because of that.

During the interview Russell examined Colin's hands, noting a cut on the knuckle of his right-hand fourth finger. He asked how it happened. Colin replied, 'It happened when I was doing the gardening yesterday, I hit a steel spike, the garden hose reel thing.'

Police obtained a search warrant for the house and both Colin and Keith agreed to be present. The search took almost four hours and various exhibits were removed, including blood samples from the floor. At one stage Russell noticed that Colin was wearing a watch with a leather band, and asked to look at it. There was some discoloration on the band and small stains on the edge of the glass face and back. The scientific officer took the watch to swab it for any potential blood, and thought the stains were likely to be blood. This was good news, for if we got the watch tested at the laboratory and the blood came back as Donna's we would have enough evidence for a charge of murder. Unfortunately we knew that getting results could take weeks.

A wallet belonging to Donna was found under the bed in Keith's bedroom; Keith said we would find it there because she left it at his place five or six weeks earlier and he had hidden it under the bed out of spite. In respect to the blood samples on the floor, both brothers said they had cut their fingers – Colin the previous day, and Keith a week before.

Both Keith and Colin agreed to give blood samples so we took them to Auburn Hospital. While we were there I asked the doctor to examine Colin's hands. His right hand was noticeably more swollen than the left and the doctor also pointed out a cut above the knuckle of the fourth finger which, in his opinion, was a couple of days old.

I asked Colin, 'Are you left- or right-handed?'

He said, 'Right.'

On a finger of that same hand Colin had a plain rectangular ring which we took for DNA testing.

It was 11.30pm when I got home after an operational briefing and paperwork. I had just finished a twenty-four-hour shift on about an hour's sleep. I was shattered. I think I just fell into bed that night, knowing I had to start again at eight the next morning.

The next day Friday 5 November was busy. We had numerous avenues of inquiry, including finding witnesses to corroborate the movements of Donna Wheeler and Keith and Colin Bond. Dr Alan Cala, who I had met in connection with the De Gruchy murders, performed a postmortem on Donna's body. He found that she had gross fracturing of facial bones with complete disarticulation and gross fragmentation of the cheekbone, two fractures of the lower jaw and a fracture of the hyoid bone. He believed that great or extreme force would have been necessary to inflict these injuries, and the attacker could have used his fists, feet or knees. He also found three stab wounds in the left chest, one of which had passed into the lung and two had penetrated ribs. There was a stab wound in the abdomen, but an absence of abdominal bleeding suggested that Donna had already been dead, or almost dead, when that wound was inflicted. Petechial haemorrhages (marks where small blood vessels had burst) on Donna's eyelids suggested that her attacker had used his hands, fingers or elbow on her neck. Dr Cala found the cause of Donna's death to be a combination of the severe head trauma and the stab wounds penetrating the left lung. There was no evidence of sexual intercourse, even though Donna had been found naked from the waist down.

A few days later Russell and I went to the morgue to see Dr Cala and view Donna's body. I was shocked to see her face had taken on a purplish colour from the injuries and bruising. This was an image I later had no trouble remembering. Her face and how the damage had occurred would later come back to affect my life significantly. I recall Dr Cala saying there was a possibility that Donna could have died from her facial injuries alone. I had difficulty comprehending that a life could be taken so easily without a weapon but simply a fist to the face. And Colin had already done this to another person.

While I was looking at her body, I noticed two small parallel cuts on her left cheek. They were a very similar size and shape as to the ring Colin had been wearing that day. Unfortunately, they were not sufficiently similar to be used in evidence but it did highlight to us that Colin was looking more like the main suspect.

The alibis given by Colin and Keith Bond needed to be tested, and the information had to be precise. On the evening of Tuesday 2 November Donna and Colin had been at the Regents Park Bowling Club intending to have a meal. James,

Donna's former partner and the father of her son, told us he had telephoned Donna that evening and arranged to meet her at Ashfield at 8.30pm. Donna had then driven Colin to the Regents Park Hotel before going on to Ashfield. While she was with James, she had arranged to pick up her son the following afternoon.

After their meeting Donna drove back to the hotel and met Colin again, around 9pm. They bought a takeaway Chinese meal at the hotel and drove to Donna's house. No witness except Colin saw Donna alive after she left the hotel with the food. Her phone records showed that she had been telephoned at 8.33pm and 8.39pm, but calls after that had gone unanswered.

We could prove that Colin had lied in the initial interview with police, and that he was also the last person to see her alive. We knew that he had been washing his clothes very late at night on the evening of 2 November, and that he had an injury to his right hand consistent with punching someone. We also saw that there were no signs of any forced entry to Donna's home. But still we did not have enough evidence to charge Colin with murder.

At last some positive results started coming in. A bloody fingerprint on the plastic bag next to Donna's head belonged to Colin Bond, and the blood was Donna's. Blood on a towel in the lounge room matched that of both Donna and Colin; this was consistent with him wiping his hands on the towel after hitting her. Donna's blood was also found on the face of the watch that Colin had been wearing that night.

Colin was reinterviewed on 15 November. When he was asked about his movements from 9.30pm to 10.30pm he said, 'Dunno, I have to, to get me, get me barrister in.' He refused to answer any further questions and was then charged with the murder of Donna Wheeler.

In June 2001 Colin Bond was tried at the NSW Supreme Court. Keith Bond was subpoenaed to give evidence but refused to attend and could not be found. He obviously didn't want to give evidence against his brother, and this gave the defence a loophole. Which brother had murdered Donna Wheeler? The defence counsel tried to get the jury to believe Keith might be responsible. Evidence about Colin's previous conviction for manslaughter in very similar circumstances was not allowed to be admitted.

On 29 June Colin Bond was found guilty. The Crown prosecutor Barry Newport requested that the jury remain to hear Colin's criminal history. It was interesting to watch the faces of the jury as they heard, in some detail, exactly what Colin had done to his previous victim in 1987.

Colin Bond was sentenced to thirty years' imprisonment with a non-parole period of twenty-five years. He died of a heart attack at Lithgow Correctional Centre a few years after his imprisonment.

After the investigation into the murder of Donna Wheeler, I noticed a marked difference in the way I perceived the world. I lost perspective about the huge significance of one human being taking the life of another, and started to view murder almost as a petty crime, like shoplifting. While I knew this was wrong and felt odd, my reaction was beyond my control. I found myself becoming more and more distanced from my emotions. I didn't feel able to trust my peers with this fundamental change. I couldn't comprehend what was happening to me and so just continued to work harder.

On my days off I tried to spend as much quality time with Jake as possible. I found that the more I experienced that love and closeness and the joy of just being with him, the more I would be possessed with negative thoughts: What if he were kidnapped? What if something awful happened to him? I couldn't turn off images of Jake in the clutches of faceless kidnappers; Jake alone and crying, and me wanting to tell the kidnappers what to do for him, even what nappies to buy, so he would stop crying and wouldn't annoy them. I kept having flashbacks of Andy's body, bruised at the hands of his kidnappers (see Chapter 9). These turned to images of Jake being hit and screamed at. These were thoughts I would never tell anyone at work as I didn't want to appear weak and was afraid they would think I was losing the plot. Maybe I was.

To try and stop thinking like this I started planning what I would do in case any of these things happened. I decided whom I would call, who would be in the police team I wanted to investigate my son's kidnapping. At least while I lay in bed crying my eyes out at the prospect of all this I wasn't seeing awful images in my head.

New challenges

At last I was able to take up my new job, promoted out of Homicide to be the investigations manager in charge of detectives at Kogarah Local Area Command. The Kogarah Local Area Command (LAC) in the southern suburbs of Sydney runs from the international airport to the southern border of the Georges River. The eastern border is the Botany Bay foreshore, the western limit is the suburb of Kingsgrove. This LAC services the Rockdale and Kogarah councils and more than 144,000 people living in this area.

I was responsible for the overall management of all the LAC's criminal investigations and for the supervision of all investigators. The staff consisted of eighteen officers with varying degrees of experience, including designated detectives and trainee investigators. We covered everything from fraud, drugs, sexual assault and robbery to murder. The job included being a senior advisor in all aspects of investigations, major and minor, and future resources planning. I was also required to take charge of any major criminal investigations. I retained my negotiator role but this promotion would involve less overtime, and my travel to and from work was considerably lessened as I was closer to home. It was also highly unlikely that I would have to travel interstate.

I also had fully sanctioned secondary employment as a consultant, approved by the NSW Police, to deliver training lectures to the staff of various companies and councils including child care, council rangers, call-centre workers and insurance company staff on various aspects of negotiation, including conflict resolution, dealing with difficult people and handling aggressive behaviour, negotiation and crisis management. This work was sporadic but I enjoyed it because I found it rewarding to see people gaining confidence in their ability to communicate. I also found delivering these lectures a kind of lifeline, reinforcing correct behaviour for me. For a time at least they helped me to cope with what I was going through.

In March 2000 I went on an in-service course dealing with critical incident investigation management. A critical incident involves death or injury resulting from the discharge of a police firearm, a police operation, a person in custody or police pursuit. The NSW Police has a mandatory set of protocols for these situations, all of which are independently investigated and overseen by the Professional Standards Command. I was especially keen to do this course, having been involved in only one Critical Incident Investigation Team (CIIT), in 1996 while I was working at the Homicide Unit (see Chapter 9).

During the day there were a variety of lectures, then after lunch we were to be given a practical exercise to test what we had learned. Just prior to lunch I was told there had been a shooting at Carlton, where a police officer had shot at a suspect who drove his car at him. I was to be the senior investigator required to set up the CIIT.

'No problem,' I said. 'Will this exercise begin straight after lunch?' Then I was told this was no exercise, but a real critical incident investigation. My office had been advised and I would see them at the scene.

I couldn't believe it. I hadn't even finished the CIIT course and here I was about to be thrown in the deep end. Incredible! This was going to be a very challenging afternoon. At least I had been given a copy of the guidelines and my Kogarah team of detectives were very professional.

A group of police from another area had tried to arrest a man who was wanted for numerous firearm and robbery offences. One officer had fired at him as he drove at the officer in a stolen car. The man had managed to escape but it was not known whether he was injured. The crime scene was secured and we interviewed all police and witnesses involved, then we had to focus on finding the offender.

He was definitely doing his best to evade police. His mother denied seeing him or knowing where he was, as I had expected she would. I asked her to pass on a message to contact me at Kogarah if she heard from him. Some days later, while he was still on the run, he rang me. The police bullet had not injured him but he declined to hand himself in. I pointed out the dangers of him potentially hitting someone but he seemed to think he was a Formula One driver and he had obviously watched too many movies like *Fast and Furious*. Some weeks later he was finally arrested and I interviewed and charged him for trying to run down a police officer. The subsequent police investigation found that the police officer had used his weapon responsibly in the circumstances.

I never did receive a certificate for completing the course.

My second callout came three months later. On 4 June two police from the Intelligence Response Team (IRT) based at Sutherland arrested a violent criminal named Christopher Edwards. Initially being refused bail, Edwards was later granted conditional bail at court. The police were told that Edwards was standing over people and had a gun. On 7 June police saw him in a stolen car at Engadine and attempted to pull him over. Edwards stopped, started to reverse his vehicle at the police then accelerated forward and drove off. Police pursued him to Old Bush Road where he jumped out of the moving car and ran into bushland. When the car stopped police arrested a female passenger and found a bag containing a shortened .22 calibre air rifle and documents in Edwards's name. A major manhunt ensued, involving the police dog squad and a police helicopter.

About three that afternoon Edwards robbed a shop owner of the keys to his Holden Calais behind the Heathcote public school. A witness quickly contacted police and members of the IRT quickly raced towards the car park.

One of these officers, Detective Smith, saw children in their school uniforms spilling out on the roadway just around the corner, then his attention was drawn to a woman in a Green Prado who was honking her horn, perhaps wanting to draw attention to Edwards's dangerous driving. He then identified Edwards in a V8 Calais accelerating sharply towards him, wheels spinning. Dust and gravel were flying. The schoolchildren were in some danger now. Smith got out of his car and ran towards the rear of the Calais, yelling for Edwards to get out of the car.

Edwards looked into the eyes of Detective Smith and reversed straight towards him, leaving Smith in no doubt that

Edwards intended to run him down. He dived out of the path of the car but a corner of the car hit him and he lost his balance. Fortunately it didn't knock him over. Smith had to make a quick calculation. He was not only fearful for his own safety but for the safety of the schoolchildren nearby, and the woman in the green Prado, who might have had children in her own car.

He drew his Glock pistol and fired one shot into a front tyre of the Calais. The tyre deflated immediately. However, this did not stop the car and Edwards continued reversing. He collided with another car which in turn was pushed into a third, causing Detective Smith to jump out of the way a second time.

Another police officer on the other side of the Calais lost sight of both Detective Smith and another IRT member who was behind Edwards's car. Fearing that they could be trapped by the Calais or fall underneath it and be seriously hurt, and mindful of the schoolchildren, he fired his pistol ten times into the bonnet of Edwards's car. The Calais stopped, being jammed up against a police sedan, and Edwards was arrested. The bullets fired into the engine did not disable it; though the car looked like something out of a Mafia shootout, it was still driveable.

Kogarah LAC was asked to investigate the whole incident as per the CIIT protocols, as one police officer had been injured and eleven shots fired towards a violent offender right outside a primary school just on school finishing time. Again I was the senior investigator. It was very clear that neither officer had wanted to shoot Edwards, even though all their training had told them to do so if there was no other way of dealing with the situation. Police are only allowed to fire their weapons if there is an immediate risk to their lives or those of others, or the risk of serious injury. In this case, I could see that the two police quite simply did not want to have anyone's death on their conscience.

After a five-month detailed investigation I formally found that they were both justified in using their firearms, though the officer who had fired into the bonnet of the car needed to have refresher training in the disciplined use of his. Even though this was only my second investigation, my report was treated and recognised as best practice in the Georges River region.

That first year at Kogarah LAC, while I still felt distant emotionally, I had new challenges that kept me busy. To aid in my negotiation training I completed a Graduate Certificate in Dispute Resolution at the University of Technology, Sydney. The highlight of this year was, of course, the Sydney Olympics and Sydney was ramping up its security measures. All police leave was cancelled during this period.

I was team leader for one of only five high-risk counterterrorist project negotiation teams. I was very proud of this, being not only the youngest at the age of thirty-two but also the only female CT team leader in NSW for the Sydney Olympics. Because of this I went to another counter-terrorist negotiators' course, this time in Perth.

In the twelve months prior to the Sydney Olympics, three national exercises (NATEX) were held, involving more than 500 personnel from state and Commonwealth agencies, including police trained in counter-terrorism from various NSW areas, the Australian Defence Force including the Special Air Service (SAS), NSW Emergency Services, Commonwealth government ministers, the NSW Premier's Department, NSW Olympic agencies and the Australian Federal Police. I took part in two of these. The exercises were held over three days and two nights, and my team had responsibility for the night shifts. Blue Ring, the first exercise in November 1999, involved terrorists taking over a ship at Circular Quay, Sydney, where IOC delegates were conducting a meeting. Ring True held in May 2000 involved forty hostages being seized by six armed terrorists during a baseball game at the Sydney Olympic Park baseball stadium. At the end of this exercise, the SAS Black Hawk helicopters were involved in a tactical resolution.

We treated the exercises as real situations, utilising the negotiators' truck and being given simulated briefings from ASIO. Operation and Tactical commanders monitored my primary negotiator conversations with the terrorists. Even though these were mock exercises, the stress levels inside the truck were intense; according to the script hostages were being shot and wounded, perhaps even killed. It was my role to monitor and manage my team, organise a time out if I felt the primary negotiator needed a break to collect his thoughts or if I considered the need to regroup the team to discuss additional intelligence and re-strategise for the next session. At the same time I was deciphering intelligence, liaising with the Tactical commander and negotiation coordinator and formulating negotiation strategies, using the help of a psychiatrist when required. Even though we were on duty for twelve hours it felt like less than half that time. After all this training, by the time the Sydney Olympics took place I felt very comfortable going into any situation.

In September and October 2000, during the Olympics and ParaOlympics, I was working full time as a CT negotiator. There were five negotiation teams, and we rotated between Sydney City and Homebush. We could access areas including the athletes' village and various events. I loved the buzz and excitement in the village as elite athletes came together to compete from all over the world. We were fortunate and so was Sydney: the only incidents consisted of political demonstrations.

After the Olympics it was time for me to return to Kogarah. In our detectives' office we had major staffing issues, as did most others around the state. Although we had a number of young trainee investigators, there were virtually no senior investigators, as they had been absorbed by various task forces. Those we did have were constantly overloaded so we had to be mindful not to burn them out: not an easy task. With other investigations managers in our region, we formulated a plan to call upon police from within our region in the initial stages of a Homicide investigation or other major incident. Even if they could come in for only a couple of shifts, that would help.

On 6 February 2001 I completed my normal ten-hour shift at Kogarah and went home to Rob and Jake. It had been a hot and humid few days, fairly typical February weather for Sydney. Just after 8pm I was called out to investigate the murder of an unidentified woman in a unit block at Kogarah. When the details had been confirmed, the rest of the office at Kogarah LAC was called out and the Homicide and Serial Violent Crime Agency were notified. The additional expertise was very welcome.

The adoptive parents of the man who leased the unit, twenty-year-old Nathan Kerr, had found the body. They had come to see him, not having heard from him for some days. They looked in through a window into the unit and saw a body lying on the floor. They broke in and were greeted by a horrific sight, but the body was a woman's, not that of their son. The police were then called.

After a quick briefing with my investigators we travelled to the crime scene. My role was to coordinate the investigation and resources. I organised for police teams to canvass the surrounding area and for statements to be taken from various witnesses, including Nathan Kerr's parents. Nathan Kerr's name was circulated via the police network as being a suspect and wanted for interview. Crime-scene officers conducted their examination.

We had a breakthrough almost immediately. Nathan Kerr had been arrested for drug offences and was in custody at Parramatta police station about thirty minutes from Kogarah. This was excellent news which needed to be acted upon immediately. The commander of Kogarah, who had turned up at the scene, reminded me of the document I had signed only a week earlier. I was three months pregnant – unexpectedly – with my second child, and had just signed off on my alternative duties agreement, which meant that I couldn't interview Kerr. I couldn't even sit in on the interview with Kerr in case he went berserk. I could, however, still continue all my management and investigation tasks, including directly overseeing all investigations.

This was frustrating, but I needed to organise a lead investigator, and quickly. One of my relieving detective sergeants, Andrew Marks, known as Marksy, was more than happy to take charge as the senior investigator and was very proficient in this role. The Homicide police and additional investigators from Kogarah would work with him.

The interview team went to Parramatta while the rest of the investigators remained at Kogarah. I chose to stay at the scene and wait for the crime-scene officers to finish their examination and to complete a walk-through of the scene with these officers and the forensic pathologist. I would give any information gathered about this to the investigators interviewing the suspect Kerr.

The smell in the unit was the usual awful overpowering stench of rancid meat and sweetish blood. The body of the woman, still unidentified at this stage, showed signs of massive blood loss and had obviously lain on the floor of the small two-bedroom unit for a couple of days. The stench was made worse by the humid weather and the fact that the doors and windows to the unit had been closed up. I had a heightened sense of smell thanks to my pregnancy hormones and every time the door to the unit was opened I became quite nauseated. I dreaded having to enter the unit as I was not sure whether my stomach would hold out.

The officer in charge of the crime scene investigators noticed my discomfort and handed me a very strong-smelling substance – a product with the inaccurate name of Nil Odour – to put near my nose. It was not quite enough to disguise the smell of death completely, but it definitely helped.

Finally it was time to enter the unit. I saw the body of a slightly built woman with long dark hair lying face down, a large carving knife sticking out from her back and a large pool of blood around her head. She had been hit over the head at least eight times with a blunt object, and this was the major cause of death. A large black Maglite torch found in the unit was later confirmed as the murder weapon. Every police car carried the same black torch, such an innocuous item apparently, but the damage it had inflicted was devastating.

The body had two stab wounds, one to her central abdomen and about sixteen centimetres long, the other on her back. The knife had penetrated her ribs and lower left lung. The forensic pathologist believed that she might have been dying or already dead when she was stabbed. There was no evidence of sexual assault.

I gave the interview team the information I now had. They told me they were still unsuccessful. Kerr wasn't saying anything so orders were under way to obtain DNA samples of his hair, hand swabs, fingernail scrapings, and photographs. There was not enough evidence to charge him with murder at this point; the investigation still had a long way to go.

We hadn't found any identifying documentation on the woman. We didn't know who she was so her fingerprints were taken in an effort to identify her. We also ran computer searches for missing persons and organised for police radio messages with her description to be circulated throughout Sydney. The fingerprint examination came back positive and we had a name, Michelle Miller, a sex worker from Kings Cross.

It was now imperative to start canvassing the Kings Cross area to see whether we could obtain any information about Michelle's last movements; where she had been, who had last seen her. Perhaps another sex worker had seen her leave with Nathan Kerr or someone else. We needed additional investigators at this stage as the team had been working all night. One of the lead interviewers waiting for the DNA samples to be taken was so tired that he fell asleep sitting in a chair and was only woken when other investigators noticed him dribbling down his tie. We had previously supplied investigators to other stations when help had been requested, and now it was our turn. Without hesitation, the other stations supplied the manpower to assist us with the urgent canvassing inquiries.

We also needed to hold a media briefing to request information from the public. Rob was the duty officer at Kogarah that morning, so he would be fronting the media. I was still at work and Rob had been late as he had to take Jake to child care, something I would normally do on my way to work. Fortunately the boss was sympathetic to our situation. I spoke with the media unit and then briefed Rob for his interview when he arrived at work.

By 11am I was starting to feel adrenalin withdrawal: I had been awake for almost thirty hours. I was due back at work that night, along with the rest of the investigators. It was time to go and get some sleep.

Over the next few days we learned that Michelle Miller had last been seen in Kings Cross at about 2.40am on Monday 5 February. Nathan Kerr had been seen on CCTV footage getting on a train at Kogarah about 11.27pm on Sunday 4 February and arriving at King's Cross railway station at 12.02am on the Monday.

We also found out that Kerr had visited his biological father, as distinct from his adoptive father, who had found the body in his unit. He had asked his father whether he knew of any prostitutes who would not be missed if they disappeared; a bizarre question. He returned to his father's home the next day and examined a law book belonging to his father; Kerr's fingerprints were found on the page describing mental health issues as a possible defence for homicide.

By 15 February enough evidence had been gathered for a strong circumstantial case against Nathan Kerr. He was arrested, declined to be interviewed and was charged with the murder of Michelle Miller.

At the Supreme Court he pleaded not guilty, citing mental health problems. He outlined a history of thought disorder, delusions of control and intrusive behaviour. He stated he had been diagnosed with schizophrenia and that a few days before the murder he had contacted the mental health service at St George Hospital Kogarah, wanting a further assessment. He reported problems with clarity of thinking, difficulties with interpersonal relationships and social contacts. He described thoughts of suicide and homicide, though denying he had any particular intention to kill himself or anyone else. He was not taking the medication he had been prescribed for schizophrenia. He had been due to attend an assessment on 2 February, three days before Michelle Miller's murder. He did not keep the appointment.

Kerr told psychiatrists that on the night of the murder he had engaged the services of Michelle Miller at Kings Cross. They had taken a taxi back to his place and both inhaled amphetamine. He said that he was very paranoid and believed that Michelle had been sent by Satan to get him killed. He took a heavy torch and hit her a number of times about the head, and then he took a large carving knife and stabbed her twice. He ran away because he thought there were ghosts and it was 'too scary' to return.

Psychiatrists who interviewed him believed that at the time Michelle Miller was murdered Nathan Kerr was suffering from an acute exacerbation of schizophrenia (the use of amphetamines was known to cause this), which affected his ability to know that his behaviour was morally wrong. The judge decreed Nathan Kerr be found not guilty due to mental illness. He was detained in a psychiatric hospital to be referred to the Mental Health Review Tribunal. If this tribunal was satisfied he was no longer a danger to himself or anyone else, he could be released.

This was a very sad state of affairs for the family of Michelle Miller. The result was also intriguing because of the evidence we had gathered concerning the law book and conversations with Kerr's father. Was he smart enough to fool the psychiatrists? As he was housed in a psychiatric hospital at the time of writing, we may never know.

CHAPTER
17

The price of making a difference

After the Michelle Miller murder I was even more on edge. I was irritable, still suffering from intrusive thoughts in relation to Jake, while at the same time feeling emotionally distant. Rob and I were arguing constantly. Rob had attended some horrific crime scenes and this was starting to affect him and our family. I think my capacity to take in any more violence and horror had almost been reached and I was struggling with what was already loaded in my memory.

Over the years, the accumulation of all the trauma and horrific crime scenes I had encountered were continuing to fill my head, like water in a sponge. Having no respite but continuing to work hard never allowed me to rest, or remove any of these shocking scenes from my mind. I didn't realise that if I continued the way I was, the sponge would become saturated, unable to absorb any more memories and horror, and its contents would ooze out and impact on all other aspects of my life. I was on a downward spiral and didn't have the foresight to recognise it.

I felt enormously protective towards Jake still. Though my second pregnancy had not been planned, I hoped that having another child would cause the scenes of horror in my mind to fade; I would be busy with two. In fact I was wishing this would be the case. Surely with two children my overprotective feelings towards Jake would not be doubled, but shared.

Rob's and my relationship had deteriorated to the point where we were having major arguments over anything, big or small. Life at home was becoming intolerable, and I was starting to feel there was no way out. Rob had now left the State Protection Group and was working at Kogarah LAC. He was considered one of Kogarah's best duty officers because of his experience as a detective and a Tactical team leader, and he genuinely cared about his team. Like me, Rob had thought that a change from his work environment would help his emotional state, but neither of us were seeking the right help.

In March 2001, one month after the Michelle Miller murder, Rob and I attended my brother's wedding at Nelson Bay, two hours' drive north of Sydney. I was five months pregnant. Nelson Bay is beautiful and I was looking forward to a couple of days away from Sydney. Unfortunately the trip became a nightmare. On the night prior to the wedding, close family all had dinner together at the local club in town. After only a couple of drinks Rob complained of a migraine the next morning and said he couldn't make it to the exchanging of vows on the beach. That left Jake, who was now almost three years old, and myself, and I felt I was once again making excuses for Rob's behaviour. At least he turned up to the reception.

I was finding it very difficult to maintain the facade of happy families. This time I had no choice, for my brother's sake, as I was the master of ceremonies. It appeared I had become an expert at hiding my emotions.

During our two-and-a-half-hour drive back to Sydney I couldn't bring myself to speak to Rob. I was sick of the arguing, I wanted out of the marriage, I wanted peace in my life. I was also pregnant and had to consider Jake. However, by the time we arrived home I had decided I could not take Rob's mood swings any longer and I told him I was leaving him. Rob was devastated.

We both agreed that Jake would come first and Rob was welcome to see him whenever he liked, or have him when I was working and he was off. I knew Rob had nowhere to go so I took Jake and moved into my mother's home.

I sought help from a clinical psychologist. I was not worried about my own mental health, not thinking I had a problem, so I only asked for advice about our marriage and Rob's apparent mental state. The thought that I might be suffering from anything work-related did not even enter my mind; it was easy to put everything down to Rob's issues. We only told one person at work what was happening, as he knew both of us well and had guessed something was up. We were both trying to keep work and personal life separate, which was difficult when we worked at the same LAC.

Rob agreed to marriage counselling, and after six weeks I agreed to move back into the family home to give our marriage another go with help and advice from the clinical psychologist. I didn't really know how I felt about Rob at that point. Did I still love him, or was I just numb? I did know that I really wanted to try and make the marriage work, particularly for the children. Rob also genuinely expressed a desire to make the marriage work.

The next few months were a blur of marriage counselling sessions, family and work. In fact I loved going into work, it allowed me to take my mind off the problems at home. Work kept me busy and gave me focus. It was also making things worse, though I did not know it at the time.

In June 2001 there was a spate of armed robberies in the Georges River region with all evidence leading to the same gang. A strike force had been set up to which Kogarah LAC had provided investigators.

Then two things happened simultaneously. I was asked to give the general duty car crew negotiating tips after they had been to a domestic violence callout involving a married couple who had recently separated. The man had grabbed a knife and their six-week-old baby and driven off in his car before police arrived. The constable spoke to the man on his mobile phone, and the man said he would kill the baby before giving him up.

This was a high-risk situation and the type of job I thrived on. It gave me a chance to block out everything and focus on the situation at hand. Different strategies and options were going through my mind when the second event occurred. The police radio sounded with two beeps which meant urgent: 'Kogarah car, any car in the vicinity, we have an armed holdup up in progress ANZ Bank, Rocky Point Road, Ramsgate, cross street Ramsgate Road ... for any available Kogarah car ...' My gut instinct told me that this was the same gang the strike force had been set up to investigate. They were extremely dangerous, and were usually armed with machetes, screwdrivers and other weapons. We now had two critical incidents at the same time.

General duties cars quickly called onto the job, as did two vehicles containing investigators. Additional car crews advised they would circulate the area for any getaway vehicles. Although my mind was busy with possibilities the police might find when they got there, I could only monitor the radio and wait for the responding crews to report back. Both teams of investigators knew what to do if the armed holdup was still in progress, or if the offenders had left.

I returned to the high-risk domestic situation and asked the general duty crew if they knew where the man was. They could only tell me that he was in his car driving somewhere in the Sydney area. I told them to get back to my office fast so we could see what information we had and what we needed to find him as quickly as possible. I was concerned that the father's mental state might become worse if the baby started crying or screaming; the mother had told us that he was still being breastfed and also needed to take medication.

The car crew arrived with the relieving duty officer in tow. I assigned an investigating team to find out whatever they could about the father and where he might possibly go. They would check his driver's licence, car registration details, any criminal history, associates, and involvement with police. We urgently needed to contact the father again. The fact that he was mobile made it all the trickier, and the on-call negotiation team were stretched between two other jobs and therefore unavailable.

As I was eight months pregnant I decided it best not to make contact with the father in case the situation changed and I had to meet him face to face. Fortunately Detective Andrew Marks, or Marksy, was still in the office. He was switched-on, calm and had very good negotiating skills. We spoke about what he should say and I gave him some advice, telling him I would stay beside him for support. My office became the forward command post. The superintendent and the crime manager both sat on one side to watch the action while Marksy and I sat on the other.

Marksy made the call. He established rapport with the father very quickly; the man was upset because the relationship had ended and he did not have access to his baby. He and Marksy spoke for some time. We knew he was somewhere near Campsie about thirty minutes away; this was confirmed when he finally agreed to meet with Marksy. Marksy now went mobile with a team of investigators, continuing his conversation with the father while he was being driven to the address.

When Marksy returned to Kogarah LAC he said that the father had given himself up without a fight. He had just taken the baby in a fit of anger, and now understood he might consider other ways of gaining access to his child. The end result was that the baby returned to the mother unharmed but hungry.

By this stage I knew via police radio that the armed holdup had been committed by the same gang as before. All the police vehicles had circulated the area but the offenders were long gone. My investigators organised for an examination of the crime scene and for statements to be taken from witnesses and the victims and all this information was passed on to the strike force.

In July 2001, a month before I was due to give birth, I started eleven months' leave. I'd always regretted not taking extra leave at half pay when I had Jake, but financially it had not been an option; Rob and I had just bought a house. More importantly Rob really needed, and was looking forward to, a lengthy amount of time off work. This was a special time with Jake, as it would be my last time with him before the arrival of the new baby.

In August I gave birth to a beautiful baby girl, Melanie. She had the most enormous eyes, a shock of dark hair, and oh my goodness, what a voice. She certainly let us know she had arrived. Melanie also realised all my worst fears. My intense feelings of protectiveness towards Jake had now doubled with Melanie. I was responsible in every way imaginable for not one but two little beings, and at times I felt I couldn't cope.

After Jake was born I had started to have nightmares that involved me holding him and being chased by rapists, child molesters and murderers. This recurring dream had me running to a clifftop where I was cornered, and always with the same question: What could I do? If I jumped I would leave him at their mercy – I couldn't do that. Did I take him with me? That would kill us both. What was I to do? And now the dreams were back, but this time I was holding both children.

I would wake in a state of panic, sweating, my breathing all over the place. I never spoke of these dreams to anyone: I felt embarrassed and didn't understand what was happening to me. I always felt that my fears were as a result of my work and the awful things I had seen. Consequently I felt that I would just have to live with them. It never occurred to me that perhaps I was suffering a mental illness, that the early signs of post-traumatic stress disorder were manifesting itself through my thoughts, actions and even dreams.

During my time off with Melanie, I also spent more time with Jake. He was, and still is, a lovely-natured and active little boy who loved to get out exploring in the backyard. The 'terrible twos' of child development did not occur with

Jake. However, by the time he was four, we knew when he was frustrated or cranky, for his feelings showed in his face and the tension of his body. This triggered images of the De Gruchy family murders. Jake was slightly built with very dark hair and when he was angry I would immediately think, irrationally, of Matthew De Gruchy. My beautiful four-year-old son was starting to remind me of that horrific killer. I started to think: *What if my son turns out like Matthew De Gruchy? Is my family in danger?* These thoughts invaded my mind every time Jake expressed his frustration, and I shut down and emotionally distanced myself from him whenever this happened. I was fine with Jake when he was happy or sad but not when he displayed anger. I knew I was keeping him at arm's length and I didn't know what to do about it.

CHAPTER

18

The art of effective communication

Early in 2001 I had decided to apply for the job of duty officer at the rank of inspector, which carried a fifty per cent
increase in salary. This would mean being in charge of the
day-to-day running of the Local Area Command, reporting
directly to the commander. For Kogarah LAC this involved
some 170 staff, and the job was both strategic and tactical.
I enjoyed my job as a detective sergeant but was becoming
irritated because relieving duty officers persisted in calling me
at home at all hours of the day or night, asking me things
they should have known. As I am an action-oriented person,
instead of sitting around complaining I decided to do something about it.

I passed the first round of assessments. Then, as luck
would have it, I was eight months pregnant for the interview
stage. Fortunately Melanie decided to stay put and I got the

job. I was not due back at work from maternity leave until mid 2002.

In early 2002 the commander at Kogarah LAC called to speak to me. He congratulated me on winning the inspector's position at Kogarah. I was most grateful.

While I still had some time off I approached a personal trainer to assist me to return to a decent level of fitness. I knew I would be returning to shift work, as well as having two children to look after, and I needed to be fit and healthy.

In June 2002 I returned to work as an inspector. I felt very proud; I was only thirty-four and this promotion made me one of the youngest operational inspectors in the NSW Police, if not the youngest. I loved the job. It had more responsibility than my previous position but was in fact easier, probably because of my background in criminal investigation and negotiation.

One of my new portfolios was in emergency management, something I thoroughly enjoyed. This involved risk assessment or identifying potential hazards and threats to the local area, which included sections of the M5 tunnel, the international airport, major roads, the railway and a major trauma hospital. It meant looking at prevention measures, our preparedness to cope with future disasters, including training staff, our emergency response and resources. I also completed a number of emergency management courses, extra training for this portfolio. My other responsibilities included mental health and employee management.

By now Rob had won the inspector's position at Sutherland Local Area Command some twenty minutes south of Kogarah. Sometimes we worked the same shift, which was on the same police radio channel. We were very fortunate to have my mother and a good day-care centre close by for Jake and Melanie. Rob and I made a good team in some ways, and mutual respect for each other's abilities and knowledge of the high-risk nature of the work brought us together. Rob gave me advice about general policing and I returned the favour with various investigative issues.

Still, wearing a police uniform again after fourteen years in plain clothes, and coming to grips with all the gadgets, lights and sirens in the marked police car, took some getting used to. I also felt somewhat inadequate in my knowledge of officer survival techniques and lack of physical strength, having always relied on my voice and communication skills to get out of trouble. I had always depended on professional Tactical police in high-risk situations, knowing they had effective weaponry and equipment as opposed to our tiny Glocks, batons and capsicum spray. Now I was no longer working with them, and that was disconcerting too.

At the LAC I noticed how easily general duties police could be injured. They were always the first to be called out. Some police officers did not pay enough attention to safety and survival procedures and I also saw an associated lack of confidence as communicators. This apparent lack of assertiveness might have been due to sensitivity or to concern that there might be later complaints about their behaviour. I had seen this more than once when I turned up to a routine traffic stop and saw the car crew being verbally abused by the offending driver. This could be attributed to a change in the current initial police training at the academy or the way internal investigations were managed at the LAC, but it was an area I wanted to address.

My goal was to help staff build confidence in their own abilities as communicators. I believe effective communication is the key to success, whether negotiating with a suspect, talking to a victim or listening to witnesses. I have been to crime scenes where multiple offenders were yelling at police, with blood everywhere, victims screaming, and police trying to work out what happened. This is not a good situation but it can be easily resolved by taking charge through communication and working through issues methodically. In leading by example, I knew my own communication abilities would be on display.

One evening, a fight broke out at St George Hospital; a group of Middle Eastern men were brawling in the casualty department. When I arrived the atmosphere was tense. Ten or more men were lined up on one side of a walkway insisting on access to the hospital, with about eight uniformed police on the other side keeping them at bay. Both sides were eyeballing each other just waiting for someone to make a wrong move, at which point all hell would break loose.

I approached the line of Middle Eastern men and asked, 'Who is in charge of you?'

One pointed to a man at the end of the line, at the entrance of the hospital. I continued up the walkway and approached him, saying, 'I am in charge of my police and I believe you are in charge of your people. We need to talk.' He was surprisingly agreeable.

Apparently one of their friends had been taken to the hospital casualty by ambulance with serious injuries because of a fight so they wanted to see him. Emotion was still running high when hospital staff refused them entry. I explained hospital regulations and the leader agreed to go in by himself and check on their friend while the rest of the group remained outside the hospital. He assured me there would be no more problems; he had just wanted to see his friend and confirm the injuries for himself. Hospital staff agreed and there were no further problems. It was an obvious solution, and the problem proved to be easy to resolve. However, with emotional issues it can be difficult for those involved to think straight.

Another kind of emotional issue arose involving the breach of an apprehended violence order (AVO). Two days previously a man named Bill had been involved in a domestic siege, and was eventually subdued after a difficult struggle with police. He was charged with a number of offences and an AVO was taken out against him, meaning he was not allowed to be within a certain distance of his victim. However, he breached the AVO and his victim told police he was sitting on a fence in a nearby street.

Two general duties car crews were already on the way and I could tell this wasn't going to be an easy arrest. This was a man who had spent seventeen of his thirty-four years in and out of gaol. I decided to head to the scene; if it turned into a siege I would already be in a position to coordinate the response. Because of my siege management background, this was a kind of situation I found interesting.

When I arrived the general duty police had surrounded Bill, who looked as if he had been waiting for them. He stood up and took a fighter's stance. Police grabbed his arms and started marching him towards the open police caged truck. He balked a couple of times but surprised police by jumping unassisted into the back of the cage truck.

The issue now was that Bill had not been searched. He knew the system and prison craft well. Conducting a search is not only standard police procedure but common sense and experience tell you never to put a prisoner, male or female, in any vehicle without doing so (see Chapter 4). The suspect might be concealing weapons or drugs, resulting in self-harm or harm to others. There had been a recent incident when a prisoner shot himself with a concealed firearm while he was in the back of a police truck.

We now had to get Bill out of the police truck to search him. After being asked to step out of the truck a couple of times, Bill was very agitated and yelled out, 'Come and get me!'

Hands went to capsicum spray and batons, chests were pumped up; clearly the police were about to meet Bill's challenge. This was not going to end well. Bill was a wall of muscle at least 1.8 metres tall. I did not want to see anyone hurt, especially my team.

'*Stop*,' I said firmly, holding my hand palm outwards towards Bill. I walked to the back of the police truck so I could see Bill's eyes but stayed at an angle to the truck in case he lunged towards me. I looked straight at Bill, who was still very agitated and moving about the truck, and said, 'You seem to be very upset; can I ask why?'

Bill seemed surprised. He was obviously not expecting this approach. He then became teary and for the next ten minutes told me his life story. He was very upset about his life and how he had been treated; he was angry about the AVO. After he had vented we talked for a short time until he calmed down to a point where I explained the police procedures we needed to follow, including that police did not want him injured and nor did I want my police officers hurt. While still not happy he indicated he understood the process and agreed to leave the truck and be searched. He did, without fuss and was taken to the police station. It was all over within half an hour.

When I returned to the station one of the constables who had been at the scene asked me to come out to the prisoner unloading area as Bill was 'playing up'. I went out and saw the truck rocking from side to side. Bill was once again very agitated and yelling out to the police, 'Come and get me, come and get me.'

I walked up to the truck and said, 'Bill, I spoke with you earlier.' Bill stopped rocking the truck.

I said, 'You promised to behave and I promised you would not be hurt. I will stay here while you get out of the truck to ensure that happens. Do you promise to behave?'

Bill started to vent again about the AVO and the unfairness of it so we discussed that for a couple of minutes. I also said he had the option of leaving the truck voluntarily, or the police having to use force against him – in either case, I said, he would be coming out of the truck.

Bill agreed to come out peacefully, and did. I thanked him and he was taken to the charge room. I did not hear anything from Bill again in my time at Kogarah.

I have always known what an important tool communication is, and one we simply do not use enough. Of course it will not work in every circumstance, as that is the nature of policing. However, I have found that in a majority of cases people want and need to be listened to.

Ironically, it was far more difficult to apply communication skills at home than it was at work. Tension between Rob and me was still rife. One morning, however, Rob came home from a night shift and I could see he was very distressed and needed to talk.

The day before, Mother's Day, a woman who had been cycling along Captain Cook Road between Cronulla and Kurnell had disappeared. Her nine-year-old son had been devastated when she failed to turn up for Mother's Day lunch. A report had also been received of a car that had run off the road that day. Rob had not been working in the morning, but that evening he had gone into work to complete an

investigation in his own time and he spoke with relatives of
the woman. He had seen her distressed son and felt his pain.
Rob had a gut feeling that he needed to go back out to the
Cronulla/Kurnell area, particularly to the site where the car
had run off the road, to do a thorough search. He did not
believe that a possible link between the missing cyclist and
the car running off the road had been investigated thoroughly
enough.

About 2am Rob went out on his own to the area where the
car had run off the road. About 2.30am he found the coloured
cover of a bike helmet by the side of the road. He looked at
it but did not touch it. He walked 20 metres further on to
where the clearing met the bushes and made heartwrenching
discoveries; the smashed-up cycle and the broken bloodied
body of the woman cyclist, about 40 metres from where the
car left the road. Rob quickly determined that she was dead.
He was shocked and saddened and totally disgusted with the
lack of attention given to searching that area earlier in the day.
He was also concerned that the woman might have survived
if she had been given immediate medical attention; however,
later it was found that her injuries were so extensive she would
have died shortly after the accident.

We spent some time together talking through Rob's experience. I knew that articulating what was on his mind it would
help him process what had happened in some small way.
Eventually he went to get some much-needed sleep.

Later that morning the home telephone rang. It was a sergeant from Miranda asking if Rob was 'all right'. I was quite
emphatic when I said, 'No,' and that Rob was very upset and
affected by the evening's events. The sergeant asked whether
he should organise a debriefing for everyone involved. I was
dumbfounded. I couldn't believe that he needed to ask me

that question as the answer was obvious; of course he should. Later I found out that the debriefing was never held nor was counselling offered to Rob. The only time Rob was able to express his despair and horror at the situation was in his conversation with me.

After this event, Rob found it difficult to sleep and was often irritable. I was also irritable and not sleeping properly, so we were constantly fighting. We could help each other in crisis, offer support, listen actively, acknowledge feelings and explore what had happened, but our day-to-day communication was breaking down and we could barely be civil to each other.

There is another side to the communication process, one that can have a detrimental effect on both the communicator and the recipient: the delivery of a death message. There can be no more devastating news than the unexpected death of a loved one, and delivering this message is one of the most difficult duties a police officer can undertake. You know you are about to be responsible for the worst moment in someone else's life. Incredibly, there is no official training to deliver the most shocking news someone will ever receive. It is an expected role of the police officer, just part of our duties.

After sixteen years in the police force I had never delivered a death message, simply because this is a role undertaken by general duty police, not detectives. This was about to change.

In November 2002 on night shift I was called to attend a fatal motorcycle accident in the suburb of Bexley. It was after 10pm when I arrived at the accident scene. There were skid marks more than forty metres from the final resting place of the motorcycle. It appeared that the rider had hit a median strip in the middle of the road, causing him to be thrown from the motorcycle. He landed some eighteen metres away with the bike possibly flipping over once or twice. His bike helmet had not been fastened properly and was found some ten metres from his body. Where his body had lain was a large pool of blood, and his head had been very badly injured.

Ambulance officers at the scene had attempted to revive him, but his pupils remained fixed and dilated and he had no pulse. He was still in the ambulance when I arrived. I decided not to view the body, more as a protective measure for my mental health than for any other reason. It wasn't necessary, and I had seen enough death.

My responsibilities included scene preservation – ensuring perimeters had been set up to divert traffic and any onlooker – that the appropriate agencies were contacted, and that police started looking for witnesses. One witness who had been behind the motorcyclist said that the rider had been travelling at high speed before losing control and hitting the median strip. This account verified what we had seen.

One of the police guarding a perimeter radioed for me to come over. A young man was sitting forlornly on a fence and the constable said she thought he was the owner of the motorbike.

His name was Frank. He said he had lent the bike to his friend Nick earlier in the evening so Nick could visit his estranged wife. Frank thought the couple might have had an argument and wanted to know if his friend was all right. I felt terrible for this young man who did not know his friend was dead. Even though Nick's next of kin had not yet been informed, it did not seem appropriate to keep the information from his friend.

I sat down next to Frank, on a concrete fence outside a house and said, 'I am so sorry to tell you this but Nick has passed away.' He looked at me in disbelief, obviously still expecting Nick to return the motorbike. I asked whether there was anything I could do for him.

I told him I had no contact details for Nick's next of kin and asked whether he could help. He pointed straight down the road towards a block of villas and said that that was where the estranged wife, Angela, lived, in almost direct line of sight of the accident. Nick and Angela had only been separated for a couple of months and Nick's family 'did not want anything to do with her'.

My general duty sergeant had just arrived after a domestic violence call. It was not my role as duty officer to deliver a death message and, much though I would have liked to hand the responsibility to someone else, I didn't think it appropriate as I had already delivered the first one. I needed to talk to Angela before she looked out a window and saw what was happening. Frank agreed to come with us to ensure we went to the right villa. We knew this was going to be shocking news for Angela, and whether or not they had had an argument she was likely to blame herself for what had happened.

When we got to the villa two blocks away Frank stayed outside. My heart was pounding as I knocked on the door. A slim woman with long hair answered it. When she saw two police in full uniform, she looked utterly shocked.

'Hello, I am Inspector Belinda Neil, and this is Sergeant Matt Layton; we are from St George Police. Are you Angela?'

'Yes,' she said in a very small voice.

'I need to talk to you, do you mind if we come in?'

She nodded.

I asked, 'Is there anyone else here at home with you?'

'No.'

She walked towards a lounge room, looking very tense and on edge. I asked her to take a seat on the lounge chair and I sat with her. After we had confirmed that Nick was indeed her estranged husband, I said, 'I have to inform you that Nick has had a motorcycle accident. I am so sorry to tell you that he has passed away.'

I gave her a moment to let the information sink in. Just as I was about to ask if there was somebody we could call to help her, she stood up and collapsed on the ground, crying hysterically. Both Matt and I attempted to help her up and console her, but her grief was so intense I am not even sure she knew we were there.

In a highly stressful situation, you often notice unusual details. I saw that Angela's fingernails were fake and very long. At one stage I held her wrists so she could not lash out at me in her hysteria, and kept thinking she was going to claw at my face because I was the person who had broken the dreadful news and caused her whole world to collapse. I understood this possibility as everyone deals with stress differently.

After a time we managed to calm her and help her into a sitting position on the lounge where I spoke quietly with her. We could not leave her there by herself. Angela was so distressed that she could not give us any contact details for her family or for Nick's, so we asked Frank to help. We finally located a phone number for her parents and organised for them to come to the house.

When I saw their car pull up I went out to greet them and delivered the sad news. Angela's mother burst into tears and went running into the house to comfort her daughter.

Now that we knew she was being looked after we could return to the police station and find details for Nick's family, who I knew lived somewhere near Bankstown. I intended to organise for local police to deliver the news to Nick's mother.

This needed to happen quickly as I was very much aware of the problems between the family and Angela.

I called the Bankstown duty officer and gave him the address I had for Nick, who had recently moved back into his mother's home. I was just off the phone from Bankstown when another telephone call came through to me. I introduced myself and immediately received a litany of abuse from a woman who said she was Nick's sister. She was most upset that Nick's mother hadn't been contacted. They had found out through Angela's family that something awful had happened.

I explained the importance of trying to locate her mother so the distressing news could be delivered face to face and not over the telephone, and said the local Bankstown police were on the way to Nick's parents' address. She confirmed the address and added that there would be trouble: all the family members were gathering at the home and were upset because the estranged wife had been contacted first.

I have found that in some cases of homicide the victim's family needs to blame someone, anyone, for the death of their loved one, whether the justice system, or the police or anyone else. For some people this is part of the grieving process, and everybody deals with stress differently. They may take on a crusade on behalf of their loved one even though they were not close, or perhaps had nothing to do with the victim. It was not my place to judge. Nick's family in their grief were very angry towards the estranged wife and anyone, police included, would bear the brunt of it.

Nick's sister asked me whether Nick was dead. I didn't want to tell her over the phone but I saw no alternative. After confirming the address of Nick's mother, and that she was with other family members, I confirmed that Nick had died. She became hysterical and hung up on me. I called the Bankstown duty officer and explained what had happened. He agreed to accompany his car crew in case there was any trouble, and to ring me with the result.

After completing this phone call, I heard my call sign over the police radio. Apparently there had been an altercation near the scene of the fatal motorcycle accident and a police officer was calling for my assistance.

I headed back to the scene, which was fortunately only five minutes from the station. On arrival I saw the female police constable who had radioed for me, and a man standing a short distance away. As this person approached me I held my hand up and told him to stop until I had spoken with the constable. The constable told me the man was Nick's brother-in-law, and he had tried to punch her and break through the barrier to get inside the crime scene. She had a short struggle with him and finally managed to convince him to wait for me. Because he was so distressed she did not charge him with any offence, which showed great maturity on her part, I thought. She told me he didn't know what had happened and had kept asking her if Nick was dead. The constable hadn't confirmed this as she was worried about his reaction and had called for me instead.

By this stage Nick's body had been taken to St George Hospital by ambulance. The police team remained on site canvassing, obtaining statements from witnesses and examining the scene.

By now I was feeling numb, particularly after steeling myself to deliver the message that Nick had died to so many people at different times and having to respond to their different reactions. I might have maintained a calm exterior in offering my sympathies but my heart went out to them and I was starting to feel like the messenger of death.

I asked Nick's brother-in-law, who was very distressed, to sit on the brick fence outside a nearby house. He said he had come to the scene to establish for himself what had happened, after information had been passed down from the family. When I told him Nick had died, he became very upset and jumped up, wanting to break through the perimeters into the crime scene once more.

I understood that this was his way of expressing his shock and distress, and calmly explained what had happened, what the procedure would now be, and why he could not enter the scene of the accident. I made him promise not to breach the police barricade. By now I was mentally exhausted and needed a strong cup of tea and a few minutes to myself back at the station.

The Bankstown duty officer called to advise that he was outside Nick's family home. Numerous relatives had arrived and initially the situation had been quite volatile, but had since calmed down. The family were going to the hospital to view Nick's body and had let it be known that there might be trouble if Nick's estranged wife Angela was there.

I spoke to the general duty investigation team who were to meet the family at the hospital and agreed to accompany them. Before going to the hospital myself, I called my staff together and we had a quick debriefing. I also spoke with each of them to ensure they were coping with the situation, particularly those who had viewed Nick's body.

At the hospital we were directed to a special room that the staff had arranged for our meeting. Fortunately Angela was not there. The family were initially hostile and I explained what had happened and why Angela had been contacted first. We had a lengthy discussion and I answered all their questions. I could see they were now over the initial shock of the news and there was acceptance as to how the evening had unfolded, but they were understandably still very distressed. Yet again I was thankful to have a background in negotiation.

There was no need to identify Nick's body, and I advised the family against seeing it because his facial injuries were so severe. I suggested they should wait until after he had gone to the morgue; I knew the attendants would do what they could to prepare Nick's body for them to view. However, the family were not to be deterred and insisted on seeing his body: maybe they needed confirmation for themselves; perhaps they needed that closure.

We all went to the viewing area of the hospital, a small room with a glass window at one end, which had a curtain drawn across it. Once more I asked Nick's mother whether she was sure she wanted to see her son's body. She confirmed that she did. I would have preferred not to be there myself because of my own issues concerning overexposure to death, but felt the need to stay out of respect for the family.

A nurse pulled the curtain back to show Nick's body lying on a hospital trolley. His face was a dark purple colour with darker splotches from his injuries. I felt sick. Nick's sister became hysterical, as did various other family members.

On the way back to the station with the investigation crew, I felt extremely upset. It was a combination of the emotional toll of the evening's events culminating in the final viewing of the body and being present during the family's grief. It took all my strength not to break down in front of the young police constables. Instead, I asked them how they were faring and listened as they spoke about their own reactions.

When we arrived at the station, the 6am shift crew had started. The oncoming supervisor took one look at me and said, 'Are you all right?'

I nearly lost it.

'It has not been a good night,' I said. 'I've just delivered five death messages.'

Like a robot, I went through the motions and debriefed the oncoming duty officer so he had enough information for the morning meeting with the commander. I put my gun away, got changed and went down to my car, which was parked underneath the police station. Before I was even out of the driveway I had tears running uncontrollably down my face. The pent-up emotions from the previous few hours finally exploded in me and I cried and cried and cried.

When I finally arrived home, however, I reverted to robotic mode. I felt cold and emotionless, as though I was in a stupor. Jake and Melanie were asleep and they looked so peaceful. Rob was also in bed asleep. I went in and sat on the bed. I really needed to talk about what had happened, but Rob rolled away from me and told me he was trying to sleep. I changed and went to bed. It would be some days before I was finally able to speak to a friend I trusted.

CHAPTER

19

The beginning of the end

After this incident I decided to take four weeks of annual leave over December 2002 and January 2003 to spend some proper time with my children and hopefully recover from my feeling of absolute exhaustion. Rob was able to take a short break and we took the children away for a week to Jervis Bay, a two-hour drive down the south coast. It was nice to leave work and Sydney behind, even if only for a short time.

On returning to work I was asked to be relieving superintendent at my Local Area Command. Having completed emergency management training, I was also assigned the role of being local emergency operations controller (LEOCON) for the St George and Hurstville Local Area Commands. This meant co-ordinating a multi-agency response in the case of a local disaster such as a chemical spill or an explosion.

I enjoyed the job and was asked by the commander to seriously consider signing up for the leadership development program, which would lead to further relieving opportunities as a superintendent. I declined as I wished to spend more time as a duty officer, not least to make any eventual promotion more credible. Besides I was still feeling physically and mentally fragile, and had decided to work part-time until Melanie turned two.

This was a very difficult decision for me as I loved my job and found it immensely rewarding. However, I felt a decreased workload would help me overcome my tiredness and lack of concentration and perhaps allow Rob and me to sort things out. We were having major problems by this point. Not once did I think about my recurrent nightmares concerning the children and what impact they might have been having.

I was pleased when my application for part-time duties was approved. Now I had a sixty-six per cent working shift load whilst still maintaining full responsibility for my portfolios. At that time there was only one other substantive inspector working at St George LAC, with sergeants relieving in the three additional inspector positions when required. These relieving sergeants were not given the same responsibilities as substantive inspectors, as the portfolios needed consistency. Now I was required to continue my full workload but only working two-thirds of the shifts. However my personal issues were getting worse.

In 2001 the Court of Criminal Appeal overturned the 1999 conviction of Graeme Mailes for the murder of Kim Meredith, based on the question of Mailes's mental fitness during the trial. His sentence was quashed and a new trial was ordered. At a second hearing Graham Mailes was found unfit to stand trial. In February 2003 we had a third fitness hearing with Justice James Wood presiding. This time Graeme Mailes was found fit to stand trial and so he was tried at the Supreme Court in Sydney. I gave evidence at the third fitness hearing and the trial, but had difficulty remembering details of the case without referring to my police statement, duty books and other documentation. I thought this was because I had been involved in so many investigations and cases since then. It was now seven years since Kim's murder.

At his second trial Graeme Mailes was found guilty. After the verdict I was invited to join Kim's parents June and Bob Meredith at their hotel in Sydney for a drink, with the officer in charge Detective Sergeant Mark Smith. I felt so sad for June and Bob, having had to sit through the case of their daughter's murder so many times.

While we were enjoying a quiet drink June brought out a photo album that held pictures of Kim's life from babyhood through to newspaper clippings of the murder investigation and court cases. As June showed me this album and talked about her daughter, her never-ending pain and suffering were obvious. She told me she wished she could have held Kim's hand and sat with her on that cold dark evening whilst the crime-scene examination was being carried out. Her words transported me instantly back to that night and I felt torn in two. As a mother myself I understood her need to comfort her child but as a police officer I had been trained to put the preservation of the crime scene first.

By this time I was also experiencing horrific mental images of both of my children being murdered. (Even writing about Kim's murder in this book, I became upset and found it difficult to breathe.) The time I had spent with June during and after the trial had humanised Kim to the point where I could no longer emotionally distance myself from the images of her brutalised body. At work, my mind was busy enough to ignore the flashbacks and keep the images at bay, but whenever I had a quiet moment they would invade my thoughts.

To keep myself occupied, taking my mind off my own issues, I concentrated on the difficulties Rob was having. He was showing signs of aggressiveness at work. If we were on a night shift together (Rob was at the Sutherland Local Area Command which bordered my command at St George) I would meet him during the early hours of the morning, when it was quiet, and have a cup of tea with him to make sure he was all right.

On one of these occasions I left Sutherland police station at about four in the morning and decided to do a general patrol around my command's area before going back to the station. It was freezing and nothing major had happened all evening. Just as I was about to go through a green light a car drove straight through the red light in front of me. I was in a fully marked police car, for heaven's sake.

A quick registration check of the vehicle via the police radio told me that the car was not stolen but that there were warnings for firearms and drug supply offences. Also our command had recently had some drive-by shootings late at night. Fully alert, I started calling my location and my team called in to assist with stopping this car. At the same time, I was worried about Rob; he was on the same radio channel and his stress levels were already through the roof. He didn't need to listen in to my involvement in a high-risk vehicle stop.

The car pulled over to the side of the road even before I activated my revolving police lights and I let the other cars know where I was – in an isolated industrial area at the back of Brighton Le Sands where, at that time in the morning, there was virtually no traffic. The police radio was giving me information about the car, together with the warnings from one of our major task forces. I knew the other cars were not far away so I got out of my car and approached the driver's side, standing well clear of his car. My hand was on my Glock 27 .40 calibre semi automatic pistol, button unclipped and ready to pull it out if needed. My senses were so highly attuned I could feel myself trembling.

The driver, a middle-aged man, started to swear at me. Because of the warnings associated with the car, I urgently needed to see his hands to ensure he was not holding a weapon.

'Put your hands on the top of the steering wheel *now*!' I ordered.

The driver continued to mouth off. This was the last thing I needed. I was having major marriage dramas, I was not sleeping properly, and I was suffering flashbacks from previous jobs. I was wired.

'Get your fucking hands on the steering wheel *now*!'

By now my pistol was out of the holster at 45 degrees to the ground. I was so close to shooting this man. *What are you doing? Concentrate*, I told myself.

Both his hands appeared on the steering wheel and there was no more mouthing off.

'Leave your right hand on the steering wheel. Use your left hand to open the door,' I said.

He did as I asked.

'Get out of the car.'

Out of my peripheral vision I saw more blue and red revolving lights so knew my team had arrived. I re-holstered but kept my hand on my pistol, watching intently as he got out of the car and onto the footpath. His courage came back and he started to mouth off again. Unfortunately for him, he picked me on the wrong morning. Considering his attitude and the warnings, I believed he had something to hide. As soon as the male crew in the police truck turned up I asked them to conduct a full strip search. When the driver was brought back he had stopped mouthing off.

The car was also searched but nothing illegal was found. The driver was fortunate to be sent away with just a red light ticket, although further inquiries would be made with the task force.

When I got back in my car, my mind kept going over the vehicle stop. I had come very close to shooting the man, and that was not good. I was so wired; it was as if my irritability meter had been turned up to maximum power.

I rang Rob as I knew he would be worrying. He said he'd relaxed when he heard me call back on from the vehicle stop, but just before that he had already been in his police car heading in my direction. This was getting ridiculous: we were both jumpy, both on edge. Unfortunately we still didn't recognise the signs of anything worse than that.

Finally, in May 2003 after many traumatic incidents Rob took leave and was diagnosed with post-traumatic stress disorder. I felt relieved for a number of reasons. He needed the time away from work to calm down and I thought it would be good for the children to have lots of time with their father at home. With Rob at home full time, we wouldn't have the extra stress of organising childcare, and I could fully refocus on my career (I would be returning to full-time work in August). I had even spoken to a work colleague about starting a Masters in Business Administration (MBA), together with the leadership development program, as suggested by my commander, to pursue my goal of further promotion.

However, I had hugely underestimated the severity of PTSD. Home became hell. Rob was angry and irritable, even more so than usual. He was also suffering from severe depression so even though he was at home every day with the children, the running of the household was left to me. His mood fluctuations made our family environment unpredictable: I was never sure what I would come home to. I was trying to manage the house, look after the children and be a working police inspector. I simply had no time to worry about my own condition and certainly none to relax.

This did not really worry me; when I relaxed my mind would fill with vivid images of my children being stabbed in their beds. These thoughts weren't helped by having to look at the events on the police computer every day. I found myself ensuring I read everything concerning the death of children or criminal offences against them, just to be sure I could cover all possible situations involving my own children and make certain these things would never happen to them. I often became very upset reading these reports and needed to compose myself before I walked out of my office. To try and take my mind off images of my children covered in blood and stab wounds, I concentrated on what I would do if I found their killer. These homicidal thoughts were entirely inappropriate, but they distracted me from seeing the mutilated bodies of my beautiful children. There was no way I could discuss this with anyone, including Rob.

I continued my life on automatic pilot. On one occasion, driving home after an afternoon shift, I went straight through a red traffic light, only becoming aware of it when another car sounded its horn to warn me. I realised that I barely remembered driving to and from work each day, or driving around on my days off, even to do the shopping.

I was also becoming increasingly forgetful. I forgot to debrief staff after they had been to a situation involving a dead body, and I forgot to confirm the status of serious jobs that needed to be delegated to the detectives. I was irritable all the time, often over the smallest things, and I realised that each day I walked into work with the mindset: 'Bring it on'. I wanted something serious or dangerous to happen during my shift, something I could sink my teeth into, rather than sitting around doing nothing. I wanted to be kept busy. I had gone beyond the limits of self-preservation and was no longer able to judge the effect these cumulative traumas were having. I had become simply an instrument for carrying out the tasks associated with my job.

In July the commander and I discussed my continuing part-time work temporarily because of the problems I was having at home. I hated having to ask as I loved what I was doing at work and really felt that I was making positive changes. I thought I could solve my problems by working less; the reality was that continuing part-time work would never resolve my issues. However, my request was turned down and I was advised to use my eleven days of accumulated family leave if I needed to. It seemed that the commander had misinterpreted my request and had thought I wanted to work part-time permanently. As a career police officer there was no way I wanted to stay part-time, but I was too exhausted to take the issue any further.

On Saturday 2 August during the night shift I checked my internal police email and saw that Graham Mailes had been sentenced for the murder of Kim Meredith the previous day. I felt sick and empty. How could I have forgotten about the sentencing? My memory was so bad these days, I was forgetting everything. I was most upset over missing it, particularly for the sake of June and Bob Meredith. I didn't want them to think I did not care enough to attend. I now remembered seeing a missed call a few days earlier from the OIC Mark Smith; I'd forgotten to ring him back. I called him straight away and he told me that Mailes had been given a twenty-five-year maximum gaol term. I rang Bob and June.

Later that evening my sister called to say that my maternal grandfather had died. He had been sick for some time in a Coffs Harbour nursing home, so this was not unexpected, but I was still very sad. I had been quite close to Pop, spending many years running behind him on his farm in northern NSW. I think, however, my emotions were too switched off at this point to feel much more. My sister was driving our mother to Coffs Harbour the following day and had asked if I would mind her children for a few hours until their father could pick them up. Of course I would, and Rob indicated he could help me, as I didn't finish night shift until 7am.

This night shift must have been uneventful, as I cannot remember a thing about it. I arrived home in the morning and remained awake, waiting for my sister to drop off her boys. Then Rob and I had an almighty argument about minding my sister's kids, he turned on his heel, walked back to the bedroom, slamming the door behind him, and went back to bed. It was nine in the morning and I was exhausted after working all night.

Rob's attitude was just part of the problems we were having, but this time things were different. I had had enough. I couldn't take any more. I stayed awake long enough to drop off my sister's boys then I went home, for the second time told Rob I was leaving, collected the kids and some clothes and went to my mother's home. I called in sick for work that night.

The next morning, Monday 4 August, I woke up and found myself shaking all over. I was having difficulty breathing and could barely function. My forgetfulness and lack of concentration were worse than ever. I couldn't remember if I had showered, put on deodorant or even if I had eaten. My head ached continuously for the next two weeks – even Panadeine tablets had no effect. Lack of sleep was making me even more irritable, especially with my children. Without my live-in tactically trained husband I was going to bed with a torch as a weapon, in case I needed it during the night. On the Wednesday I flew to Coffs Harbour for my Pop's funeral. At the airport in Sydney, waiting to depart, all I wanted to do was scream for no apparent reason. My chest remained so tight I couldn't breathe properly.

Now I knew I had a major problem. I couldn't explain what was happening to me and it was time to seek professional advice. I started seeing Vera Auerbach, a clinical psychologist, who had provided Rob and me with marriage guidance counselling two years earlier. After analysing my symptoms and giving me a number of psychometric tests, Vera diagnosed that I was suffering from chronic post-traumatic stress disorder. My symptoms were so severe I began seeing her once or twice a week.

A dear friend who had never seen me in this state before was so worried that she drove me to a psychiatrist we both knew from work. He gave me the name of a psychiatrist at Kogarah who, on my first visit, said I must have time off and provided me with a certificate for three months of sick leave.

On Friday 15 August my commander and another duty officer visited me at my mother's home to check on my welfare. I handed over the certificate for three months' sick leave.

My commander's words were, 'They [psychiatrists] always go overboard.'

I started to explain some of my symptoms, including my forgetfulness, my irritability with the children, and snapping for no reason. My commander said that he too yelled and became irritable with his children. The duty officer told me he was also very forgetful. I reminded them of our age differences. They were both over fifty and I was thirty-five. At one stage the duty officer said, 'You don't have to put this act on in front of us.' Unfortunately, this reaction was indicative not only of the police culture but the lack of understanding of PTSD.

Later I received a call from the NSW police rehabilitation officer, whom I had previously contacted several times to organise counselling and debriefing for police involved in critical incidents. I requested that work personnel no longer contact me. I was finding it difficult enough to come to terms with my lack of functioning and I didn't want to have to explain this to someone who wasn't really listening. I just wanted to try and relax.

I was fortunate enough to have two close work colleagues who were genuine in their concern and I trusted them both implicitly. They called me and it made such a difference knowing that there were people who truly cared about my welfare.

Over the next few weeks the intermittent headaches continued. I couldn't relax, couldn't seem to turn off my mind. I still couldn't breathe properly and at times when I lay in bed it felt like someone was sitting on my chest. The nightmares were still there, and I was not sleeping well. I thought perhaps a trip away with the children might help me to relax. In September 2003 I decided to take five-year-old Jake and Melanie, aged two, away for a holiday.

Mum came along to help me cope as well as have a holiday herself. We decided to go to Daydream Island in the Whitsundays.

It looked just like the brochure; a beautiful location, gorgeous landscaping, swimming pools for the kids, and a day spa for Mum and me. Unfortunately I still couldn't relax. I was extremely hypervigilant. There was a play area for children in the restaurant and when we went for dinner I couldn't keep my eyes off Jake and Melanie for fear they would be kidnapped or disappear. I couldn't stop myself developing emergency plans, even to the point of working out where I would send staff to look for my children, which particular areas to survey, how I would organise briefings, the length of time it would take police to arrive on the island. On one windy morning I was taking a walk around the island and saw a helicopter land on the helipad near the walkway. I went straight into emergency planning mode in case the helicopter blew off the helipad due to the wind, working out how I could protect my children.

I was glad to get back from the holiday; relaxation had been so elusive. This continued, I still couldn't relax. Weekly massages, however, gave me some relief and I would normally walk out from a massage in a daze. When I took my children to a local park for a girlfriend's birthday, by the time I got home I was anxious, felt very stressed, angry and had pains in my chest, simply from trying to keep an eye on my children in the park.

I felt I was losing my children. I was always so stressed trying to protect them, my hypervigilance was exhausting me, I couldn't seem to relax and enjoy time with them. I had lost the ability to simply get down on the floor and play with them.

On my fourth visit to the psychiatrist at Kogarah I finally opened up to him about the Kim Meredith murder. I found this incredibly confronting and distressing, not having been able to bring myself to go into detail about this particular case.

After this visit my symptoms seemed to escalate. One night I managed to read Jake and Melanie a story before bed, then jumped in the shower and cried uncontrollably. I felt I couldn't cope as a mum. I knew what my capabilities were and I couldn't believe that I was getting worse. I was spending time away from work, why wasn't I feeling better?

On the day of my next appointment with the psychiatrist the receptionist called me at home to tell me he was seriously ill and would not be returning to work until the following year. I put the phone down and started to choke. I couldn't swallow and I couldn't breathe. Then I burst into tears. I had finally found the courage to talk to someone in detail about the Kim Meredith murder and now he was off sick for months! I tried walking around the house to calm myself down. I was terrified. I didn't realise it but I was suffering my first ever panic attack.

Jake was at preschool, but Melanie was home with me. I was worried about her safety in case I was having a heart attack or stroke. I rang Rob and told him to come and get her, then I put her in my mother's laundry basket. If Melanie was in the laundry basket, I reasoned, she couldn't hurt herself if I was unable to protect her. Melanie could stay there until Rob came.

I went into the kitchen, still crying uncontrollably. Vera, my clinical psychologist, had encouraged me to monitor my breathing rate using my watch. To give myself something to focus on I timed my breathing: nine breaths in ten seconds. (I was later told that fifty-four breaths in sixty seconds is considered dangerous and could lead to cardiac arrest.)

I continued timing my breathing as it allowed me to concentrate on something and I didn't know what else to do.

Rob arrived shortly after and took Melanie. I couldn't even talk to him about what was happening. What was I going to say? I didn't understand it myself. I couldn't believe my body had reacted so strongly solely because I had opened up to the psychiatrist about one particular murder.

I was still seeing Vera twice a week and I made an appointment to see yet another psychiatrist, Dr Greg Wilkins at Miranda. Unfortunately this would not be until October, over a month away.

During this month the young daughter of a dear friend and work colleague died from an aggressive cancer. I rang and spoke to my colleague's wife, I felt so helpless in not being able to give him further support, the only comfort knowing that he had good solid friends around him. I was quite simply incapable, although my own problems were so far removed in comparison to what he and his family were going through and it didn't seem right to feel the way I did. I felt paralysed and unable to emotionally connect with my dear friend. This emotional numbing, I later realised, is one of the cardinal symptoms of PTSD.

Part of my struggle was the intellectual knowledge of what was required and what was appropriate as against my seeming paralysis to communicate. This resulted in further complexity, which compounded my frustration and left me feeling perplexed and devastated that I was not able to be more of a support to my colleague.

Vera was once again counselling Rob and me about our marriage. Six weeks after our separation I had decided to return to Rob. This was the third time. Once I had been diagnosed with PTSD I wasn't sure whether my symptoms had been the cause of my decision to separate. At that time I believed that now Rob and I had both been diagnosed with PTSD and were working with the right professionals, perhaps our marriage might also be saved. We were both still struggling with our symptoms but knew why we were behaving in this way. We were also trying to support each other. When I moved back in with Rob I felt safe again.

In November 2003, we decided to take the children for a holiday to Vincentia, a lovely little town about two hours' drive south of Sydney. On the drive down I felt more relaxed than ever but as soon as I relaxed the problems started again. My thoughts flew from one crime scene to another, as if I was watching a video of all the jobs I had been to. I relived the police pursuit that had resulted in the death of Tim, my colleague at Waverley back in 1987; I saw the accident site, went to the funeral and then visited Tim's parents' home all over again. During these flashbacks I could literally 'feel' the weight in the coffin and Tim's body sliding towards me as we pallbearers walked down the church steps.

When we reached Vincentia I looked at Rob and said, 'I see dead people.'

Upon returning home after our week in Vincentia, I was more anxious than ever from trying to block out these images. My sleeplessness and breathing difficulties became worse. I was doing four or five loads of washing a day and spending hours in the shower. It felt as though I was trying to remove all the blood from my mind. I was suffering from increasing panic attacks while at the same time feeling very detached from my family, including my children. I was feeling emotionless and robotic.

Doing anything at all was an effort, a particular problem with Christmas approaching. My concentration remained poor. The bad headaches continued, along with dizziness. To try and relax, I signed up for an eight-week beginner yoga course. However, whenever we were asked to meditate I had to keep my eyes open and focus on various things in the room to stop the awful images that threatened to overwhelm me. I did not continue with yoga as I was afraid my emotions would get the better of me and I would break down during meditation in class.

On 7 December 2003 my beautiful Jake summed up my disposition in one sentence: 'Please don't be angry all the time.' I was trying not to but it was hard, very hard, and I really didn't know what to do. I *was* angry and frustrated. I didn't want to be off work. I was a career police officer and couldn't understand why my mind was behaving this way.

By now I was seeing Vera and the new psychiatrist, Greg Wilkins, three times a week. One of the first tasks Greg gave me was to sit quietly for ten minutes every day. I was to do nothing, just sit still. The first time I did this the time seemed to drag on. I checked my watch to see how much longer remained, but I had only been sitting quietly for one minute.

Christmas was imminent and I knew I had to make an effort for the children's sake. I decided to show them some Christmas lights; I enjoyed them so perhaps this would pick me up also.

'Okay, kids, who wants to go and see some pretty Christmas lights?'

'Me! Me!' the kids called out, their enthusiasm bubbling over.

It was so beautiful to see their little happy faces, such a contrast to the emptiness I felt inside. I put my robotic smile on and we drove to the street where home owners had put together sparkling displays. I opened the door for the kids.

Their eyes lit up and they ran to the first house, fingers pointing.

'Look Mummy, look!'

'Yes sweetie, Santa Claus and his reindeers,' I said. They looked as I felt, plastic, mechanical and false. The kids ran from one house to another, I followed. I barely noticed the displays as I watched the children dart from place to place. They ran, I could barely keep up. My breathing rate started to get faster. It was dark and I was worried about losing the kids in the small crowd of other children and parents.

Where were they? Ah there they were, near a musical display, with the sounds of 'Jingle bells, jingle bells...' permeating through the crowd.

'Come on kids, time to go.'

'But Mum ...'

'No buts, now!'

Back in the car I breathed a sigh of relief – I had the kids safe and we were going home.

A few days later Rob went to the gym for a workout while I stayed home with the children. They were playing with each other and then, as kids do, started annoying each other. I couldn't stand it. They were driving me nuts! Rob was due home in an hour but I couldn't wait that long. I rang Mum.

'I'm coming over with the kids.'

We stayed at Mum's for lunch and she played with the kids. I took them home later in the afternoon.

That night I was very upset. I lay in bed thinking *I can't cope with kids, what else could I do?* I felt like such an idiot.

Christmas did give me some respite as I kept myself busy with my family to try and block out the flashbacks. My short-term memory was so severely reduced that I would carry sticky notes with a list of my tasks for the day, or a list if I needed to go shopping. My skills at multitasking had also disappeared. I had been able to lead a team of negotiators, deciphering intelligence, managing the team, formulating negotiation strategies, planning tactics and liaising with the other senior members of the command team all at the same time and under incredible pressure. Now I would walk into a room and forget why I was there. This happened more than once a day.

I avoided watching the news, as on the rare occasions I did I would become extremely upset at anything involving children or death. My breathing would become more rapid and I had to try and calm myself using the breathing techniques I had been given. It felt that my ability to take on any more stories about death or injuries was saturated.

I was becoming more paranoid about my children, anxious whenever they stood in front of the glazed front windows of the house because of the possibility of a drive-by shooting. These were not uncommon in the St George area where I used to work, although amazingly nobody had been injured. I also considered the possibility that Paul Offer (see Chapter 13) might organise such a shooting from inside gaol. He had already been charged for attempting something similar. My hypervigilance and irritability made taking my children to the shopping centre or anywhere else too difficult and it was easier to stay home.

On one occasion I was involved in a road-rage incident. The car came racing out of the side street. I hit my horn and swerved to avoid it, narrowly missing a car in the next lane.

'You idiot!' I yelled, knowing he couldn't hear me but had seen me mouth the words. It was a release of frustration after he had nearly wiped out me and my two-year-old daughter sitting in her child restraint seat in the back.

I caught his look of anger then he slowed down in the lane on my right. I went cold. As he slowed down next to me I saw he had pulled out a gun, similar to a police issue semi-automatic Glock pistol. He aimed it right at me. Oh my God, I thought. Someone had once waved a screwdriver at me in a road-rage incident but never a pistol, and my daughter was in the car.

My first action was to get us out of there. I put my foot down hard on the accelerator to put some distance between us, then I heard the explosive sound of the gunshot followed by breaking glass.

I turned and looked into the back seat. The most horrific sight imaginable greeted me. My daughter was still strapped into her child restraint but blood was spraying out of her neck where her beautiful head had been. Bright red blood spurted from her neck to the roof of the car whilst her body, her arms, her legs were still strapped into the restraint. It was surreal, it was horrendous. I could very clearly see severed arteries and veins flopping around in what was left of my daughter's neck.

I looked away, turned my head again and saw that my beautiful daughter was still sitting in her seat and looking at me with a puzzled expression in her big brown eyes. It had all been an hallucination. The other driver had only been momentarily annoyed. I was sick to my stomach. I pulled over to the side of the road as it took a few minutes to collect my thoughts. I needed to get home, to familiar surroundings so I could try and recover. How much longer would this continue?

20

A dark time

By January 2004 a number of different cases I had been involved in were running through my head: Tim's fatal pursuit, the murder of Kim Meredith, the murder of Donna Wheeler, the hostage situation with Jack in Carlton. I went over and over that. I kept asking myself why I'd just stood there when Jack came at me with the knife; why had I needed to be pushed out of the way? I was still feeling very detached from everyone, and extremely paranoid about my family's safety. If Rob went to the local shops or to get a video, I would start hearing potential intruders outside the house.

In December the rehabilitation officer rang and said that the senior management team from St George LAC wanted to contact me once a month. I had been allocated a welfare officer, whose job was to conduct 'welfare checks' on me and keep in touch to see how I was progressing. My welfare officer, one of the other duty officers I had worked with, had called me twice in the previous few months but I had not heard from him after that.

He had to fill out a form each time he contacted me. I agreed to this but was still paranoid after the comment about putting on an act from the duty officer who had visited me; the commander had also told me he had needed to 'defend' me to his peers. I had always put one hundred per cent into work so I didn't understand this. Apparently I had upset the system by going off sick with a stress-related illness.

I was still angry with myself for not recognising my symptoms sooner and doing something about them. The reality was that the lack of support from work was partly my own doing as I had not told anyone about the nightmares and flashbacks I had endured for years. I had not sought help for fear I would be ridiculed. It was generally known that if you couldn't handle stressful situations as a police officer, your chances of promotion would be affected.

In January, I was very upset when I heard that someone I had trusted had told a friend of mine, 'She can be a control freak. Sometimes things don't go her way.' A reference, no doubt, to my application for part-time work being turned down. I was also insulted and hurt when a friend of Rob's imparted the news of another rumour. Someone was claiming that Rob and I were off work 'rorting the system'. The person in question had talked about 'these women who get pregnant then get pregnant again, then go off sick because they didn't get part-time leave'.

This comment highlighted to me what some senior police were thinking and how my name had been damaged. As a result I became more reclusive. I wanted nothing to do with anyone from work, I felt alone and isolated. How could they say I was rorting the system when I was going through the hell that was currently my life?

I guess these comments came from the fact that at work I was no shrinking violet; I gave my opinion when asked and never kissed anyone's backside. I often wondered whether I would have been treated differently had I been wearing a bandage wrapped round my head. General Peter Cosgrove, Australia's governor-general and the former chief of the Australian Defence Force, has described the situation best: 'You and I can see a wound or a broken bone, but an injured mind is another matter' (*Newcastle Herald*, 24 April 2013).

I bumped into the rumour-monger one day at our local shopping centre and was finally able to tell him what I thought about the comments. I didn't bother staying for a reply; I was beyond angry. I can only hope that such people have learned to keep their opinions to themselves.

More upsetting still, I think, was the comment from a former police officer whom I held in high regard. 'I thought she was stronger than that,' she said about me. This probably upset me the most because I agreed with her. I'd thought I was stronger than this too. I'd thought I could handle anything, and now I felt I had let the side down.

Even within the family, people didn't understand. A family member who is also a police officer told me he couldn't understand why I hadn't gone back to work once Rob and I decided to give our marriage another go. He was convinced I'd taken sick leave because of our marriage problems – and he didn't once ask me about my work issues or being diagnosed with PTSD by more than one highly qualified mental-health professional. This conversation reinforced my need to distance myself from others. I desperately wanted and needed support from my family and friends, but I couldn't discuss the incidents that had caused my distress. I became increasingly withdrawn.

The night after I had heard the comment about rorting the system I had a terrible nightmare. It was a dark evening and I had been called to a negotiator incident with a man at the Gap, the cliff on the South Head peninsula in Sydney's east that was infamous as a suicide location. The man was holding Melanie over the edge of the cliff. She was just a baby.

'I am here to help you,' I said. 'Why don't you put the baby down and let's talk.'

I continued to talk to the man but got no responses and I did not recognise his face. Nothing I was saying was getting through to him and Melanie was still dangling over the edge. I was terrified I would lose my baby.

He held her over the edge to taunt me. I didn't know what to do, I couldn't reach her, I couldn't reach him. I tried and I tried to talk him into letting her go.

Then he did let her go. He dropped her over the edge.

I raced forward to try and grab her and woke with a start, choking as I tried to take in air.

In January 2004, I had an appointment with an independent psychiatrist to investigate my formal claim that I had been 'hurt on duty'. The appointment involved an hour-long interview. I found it harrowing, as it once again required me to open up and discuss the various horrors I had seen. During the interview, I experienced flashbacks to Kim Meredith's body. I could see the terrible wound in her throat, the blood, the twigs and leaf litter in her hair. It was too real and horrific for me to discuss with someone I had only just met. I supplied brief details of some of the situations I had been involved in, but no more than that.

After I left this interview I was distressed that I hadn't been able to be more forthcoming, that I still had so much trouble articulating my experiences. Part of the problem stemmed from my belief that my first psychiatrist had become ill because I had opened up to him. At the time I had had a severe panic attack. I felt I needed to shield others from my experiences, particularly family and friends.

My inability to give the independent psychiatrist the right information only served to worsen the way I was feeling. He said I would only need another six to twelve months of treatment – yet here I am, many years later. He also suggested I should discontinue massages as they were not an approved method of treatment. I am not an expert but I completely disagree, as I found massage to be one of the best ways to help me relax.

In January 2004 Jake started kindergarten in a primary school catering for more than 800 students. His preschool had been a small place with security fencing; anyone who walked in was easily seen by the staff. The first thing I noticed about the new school was the dilapidated fencing, which was barely a metre high, and the lack of gates at the entrance. It was such a big school that it would take some time for anybody who walked in off the street to be officially identified.

I started imagining the possibility of a domestic violence siege occurring there – an enraged father upset over custody issues and holding Jake's class hostage. It was a possibility I had already considered at Jake's preschool, but it was worse now as he would be going to school five days a week. Another example of risk assessment gone haywire.

Vera, my clinical psychologist, had advised me to keep a diary of all events, thoughts and feelings while I was on sick leave. *I feel weird,* I wrote, *getting that really detached feeling again – is this the onset of the video flashbacks again? Feel like crying but no tears, very tired and sad. Scared of more flashbacks – feel like they are hovering above me.*

I tried visualisation and relaxation tapes, but found I couldn't concentrate on them. I was also still finding my task of sitting quietly for ten minutes extremely difficult.

On 30 January 2004 I looked in the local newspaper for kitchen advertisements as we were going to renovate our house. It was another way to keep busy. I saw the name Ivan Christov at the top of an article relating to the murder of a woman almost three weeks before. Christov had been the hostage taker during an eight-hour siege back in September 1996 at Crows Nest (Chapter 9). His hostage and ex-girlfriend Grace had beem stabbed by Christov and was lucky to be alive. Christov had murdered Lynette Phillips, a former girlfriend who had broken up with him. I read that he had tied her hands together, and also tied a shoelace and a leather dog lead around her neck. She died from asphyxiation. This was Crows Nest all over again, but this time his victim hadn't been so lucky. Just prior to the murder he had tried to run Lynette off the road. She had reported this to St George Local Area Command, where I had been working before taking sick leave.

I felt goosebumps all over my body as I read the article and I couldn't breathe. I knew Christov's background. In my confused way of thinking I believed I might have been able to prevent the murder. A panic attack set in and I began to cry uncontrollably. I felt so much guilt. If I hadn't been on sick leave, there was a one-in-five chance I could have been working on the shift when this woman came in seeking help. I knew how dangerous Christov was; I would have told her about the kidnapping in 1996, even though I was legally bound not to because of privacy laws. I started to feel responsible for her death; if I hadn't been on sick leave, I thought, she might still be alive.

I was also in shock that Christov had not been in gaol; the hostage episode had taken place only eight years before. I later discovered he had received a mere twelve months for each charge of malicious wounding (two counts), which he served concurrently. He had also received a minimum seven months, with an additional term of two years for unlawful imprisonment.

After reading this article the Christov flashbacks intensified, particularly the look of fear and distress on Grace's tear-stained face and the sight of her shirt covered in blood from the stab wounds. I remembered the feeling of total helplessness I had experienced, of knowing she was scared and in pain, but only being able to watch what was happening from the doorway to the bedroom. These feelings coursed through me day after day and compounded what I was already suffering. During February 2004, when I was walking around my house or driving in my car, I would start crying for no reason. I felt empty and sad and could not snap out of it.

Becoming more irritable and angry with kids, I wrote in my diary. *Breathing levels going up, feel teary as am not handling myself well.*

By 6 February Vera suggested that I needed time out, even a trip to hospital. No way! That was not an option for me. That would mean I was really ill and I still didn't want to believe that. Greg, my psychiatrist, had tried on a number of occasions to get me to take antidepressants, but I refused, believing I would become one of the people I used to negotiate with.

Towards the end of February 2004 I knew I needed time to myself. *Nothing is going right,* I wrote in my diary, *goal posts keep getting moved – getting harder to see the light at the end of the tunnel. Hospital not an option ... Suicide not an option – look at what is left behind, damage to family, kids, police who come etc. SELFISH ... Feel sad and empty.* I was even forgetting to eat and could go a day without realising I hadn't had any food.

Jake was getting into trouble at school. He'd been throwing sticks and stones at a fence and continued throwing stones on a school neighbour's roof after being told to stop. He was also being rude to the teachers. I blamed myself for his behaviour. My beautiful son had two parents who were irritable and angry most of the time, no wonder he was bouncing off the walls at school. I felt so guilty that he was subject to our home situation and I felt powerless to stop anything. I wanted to try and think about what was happening to me and it was getting too difficult to cope with my needs and the needs of my family with two young children and a mentally ill husband. I still didn't believe I was suffering a mental illness.

I decided to book into a health retreat and found a lovely spot in the Southern Highlands at Bundanoon called Solar Springs. It advertised 'relaxation and rejuvenation' – exactly what I needed. I booked two nights.

On Sunday 24 February 2004 I packed my bag in peace. I could hear the children playing at the front of the house and Rob talking to the neighbour in the front yard. My thoughts were filled with my need to escape. I walked out to my little green Mazda 121 parked in the driveway and put my bag in the boot, walking right past Rob and the neighbour without even acknowledging either of them. I wasn't meaning to be rude. I got in the car, started the engine and reversed out of the driveway.

'Hey!' shouted Rob, giving me a strange look.

I stopped the car. I couldn't believe it but I had forgotten to say goodbye. I had been oblivious to everything going on around me except the trip to the health retreat. I drove back in and said my goodbyes to Rob and the children.

Bundanoon was an easy hour and a half drive south west of Sydney. My room had a double bed and view over the valley. I jumped on the bed and felt ... absolutely nothing, just sheer emptiness.

The next morning there were a number of activities available but I only felt inclined to do a short bushwalk. I thought that would be perfect and relaxing. Breathing in the clean brisk air and basking in the splendour of the views of surrounding hills and forests. This was a lovely start to the day.

Our guide took us to a clifftop overlooking the Morton National Park. The view was indeed very beautiful and serene; the trees, the mountains, and the birds, so unspoilt, so peaceful. It was such a stark contrast to the jumbled chaotic mess of my mind. I was struck by the thought of the Gap, a place of beauty, tranquillity and amazing views. A place I had been called out so often to negotiate with people who wanted to commit suicide by throwing themselves from its clifftop.

I returned to my room after the bushwalk and spent the next few hours wondering why my thoughts kept wandering back to the clifftop and why I wanted to go back there. Being off work and supposedly relaxing seemed to open the floodgates of even more horrific images from crime scenes. It wasn't only the images I needed to comprehend but my associated feelings and thoughts of fear, shock, sadness, and distress that came with the pictures. These intermingled with thoughts about my inability to mother my children, my deteriorating marriage, my worsening communication skills, my forgetfulness, my lack of concentration, my irritability. I only saw my situation worsening. I did not have the distractions offered at home and I began to yearn for the calmness and serenity offered by the view from the clifftop.

Having no one I could confide in and no coverage for my mobile telephone, I took to writing in my diary whilst I was in my room. It seemed to help in processing what I was thinking as I was so confused.

Went for a walk to Grand Canyon lookout – beautiful view very calming but then drawn to clifftop, think Gap. Could be easy way to do it – can't believe thoughts that come into your mind, it's like a constant struggle as I am not going to do anything but thoughts keep coming (eg jumping off cliff easier than fixing up exhaust).

Why do the thoughts keep coming? It is becoming automatic? Now the worry is not just about kids' safety, it is like I am also concentrating on mine but I have no intention of doing anything, it is scary, need to ask more questions and things about future – need positive things, feel at rock bottom. WHAT DO I WANT TO DO? I DON'T KNOW ANYMORE. Feelings of sadness, nothing.

Pedicure – Fabulous – then paraffin wax and skin looks eerie; beautician says she was asked if it was like a dead person's. I CANNOT GET AWAY FROM IT.

I continue to have thoughts about the Grand Canyon. I want to go back down but have yoga at 4.30 – Why do I want to go down. I don't know, it was very breathtaking, so is it the scenery or other. IS THIS ALL JUST A BAD DREAM & I WILL WAKE UP. If I am at home I am busy with kids I don't

have time for these thoughts but then am getting too busy.
(Yoga 4.30 teary during same & relaxation at end).

Looking back on this, it was as if I was using my negotiating skills to save my own life. I was negotiating with myself. My thoughts drifted from the calmness and the serenity I viewed from the clifftop to my muddled, confused mind. I wanted to be part of that calmness so badly that it was frightening. I wanted so much to be free from the emotions and symptoms I had been experiencing; the sadness; the feeling of detachment from my children and people in general; the irritability; the hypervigilance; the forgetfulness; the lack of concentration; the lack of sleep. My diary was my only way of getting the thoughts out of my head to seek relief and make sense of the mess in my mind.

It was as if I was living two lives. On one hand I would leave my room and attend every meal, sitting with the same four people and taking part in conversations. Then I would return to my room and think and write the way I was feeling in my diary. I was trying to maintain normality whilst struggling with a solution that I would never, in normal circumstances, have contemplated. A yoga class or having a pedicure was like an anchor in a brewing storm. In a sense I was still looking after myself but when in my room, the thoughts would come flooding in. When I was busy I seemed to cope but as soon as I was alone my mind wandered into darker realms. I felt so alone.

That night my thoughts continued to drift to the clifftop. The pressure to return was immense. I was fighting with myself. I continued to ask myself the question: *Why do you want to go there?*

I knew the answer, but couldn't bring myself to say it or write it. My thoughts drifted to Rob and the children, but not as a reason *not* to go back to the clifftop. Instead, I found myself composing a suicide note. In my distressed state of mind, I believed that a piece of paper with the word 'Sorry' and three 'Xs' placed on the dashboard of my car, parked near the clifftop, would answer their questions. It became a struggle to think of anything beyond whether I should go back there or not. I knew in my heart that if I did I would never return.

Again I began negotiating with myself and conducting a risk assessment. What if I jumped off the cliff and didn't die? What if I got caught in the tops of the trees, injured, dangling from the branches? What if I had to be rescued? Everyone would know I had tried to commit suicide. How would I explain that? And if I died, what about the police who would need to come to the scene? They didn't need to go through that. These thoughts did stop me going to the clifftop.

I found a public telephone box near reception and rang home. Rob asked if I was okay and of course I said I was fine, just as I would smile when I went into work every day. A smile hides everything. It felt calming, though, to hear his voice. I was able to go back to my room and the thoughts calmed down somewhat.

On my last morning at Solar Springs I woke up with the same thoughts in my head. I had to drive home today, or would I drive to the clifftop? I felt nervous and undecided. I was almost scared to get into my car. I need to do something and keep busy. I went to a shiatsu massage demonstration then it was time to go home to my family.

On the drive home along the Hume Highway all I could think about was how close I had come to wanting to end it all, how little I had thought of my children as my mind was in such a mess. This was the first time in my life that I had ever considered suicide. I had never thought I would feel like this. I felt embarrassed and confused. I didn't know myself any more.

I had once considered suicide to be a selfish act, but when it came down to it I had spent the previous evening struggling with myself. I truly believe that a person just gets beyond the point of logical thinking. To have someone intervene at that point and to have someone to talk to is so important to help sort through the confusion. Being a negotiator I had never fully perceived suicide from the mind of someone wanting to commit it. Now I felt I understood the mental state of someone in this position.

All I needed was someone to talk to, someone I could rely on, but they all seemed so few and far between. Two of my dearest girlfriends were also struggling with PTSD and I didn't want to burden them with my problems. My other dear friend was a schoolteacher and beautiful person, but I couldn't bring myself to tell her how bad it was. If I had told these friends what was happening, I know full well they would have dropped everything to help me. All I wanted was to get back to Sydney and throw myself at the mercy of my mental-health professionals.

CHAPTER
21

Acceptance

At the end of February 2004, after I returned from Solar Springs, I walked into my psychiatrist Greg's office with my hands outstretched in front of me, as if I was waiting to be handcuffed, and said, 'Okay. I guess a hospital visit is in order.'

I knew I had overstepped an emotional boundary in coming so close to committing suicide. Meeting with Greg that day I did not feel that I was giving in, just relieved at having decided to put my life in someone else's hands. To let someone else take total control. I had finally accepted that I needed help, even if that meant admission to a psychiatric hospital, the use of antidepressants and anything else Greg recommended.

I confessed everything to him, including my fears of how close I believed I had come to killing myself. At that moment I no longer had any faith in myself or my decisionmaking.

To my total surprise Greg advised me that even though I was severely 'impacted with' PTSD, I was at the point where I had finally accepted this condition and so there was no need for me to be admitted to hospital. I had demonstrated to him that I was capable of getting better and I needed a degree of autonomy. He and I would work together to an established plan, which involved appropriate medication and psychotherapy. This also included an emergency plan should I relapse.

In a nutshell, I was on a short leash. I experienced overwhelming relief after discussing what had happened and why, including the plan I was now to follow. This plan gave confidence back in my own ability to help myself, albeit I would be taking the antidepressant Zoloft. There was no more arguing from me on that point. I also made the decision not to go near any cliffs as I didn't trust myself any more and decided it wasn't worth the risk.

The antidepressant medication, which I had initially fought so hard not to take, was prescribed because I was overwhelmed by so many raw emotions and it assisted in deadening emotional reactivity. It numbed my reactions to unpleasant things, and I wasn't as upset. I still felt sad but I couldn't cry. However, it also served to numb me from experiencing enjoyable emotions such as a hug from my children: this was the trade-off. I didn't feel as angry or disturbed but I didn't feel joy or happiness either.

At one stage my Zoloft was increased to 75mg a day. I felt as though I was in a dream-like state. I found that in conversations with friends I would be at least thirty seconds behind the conversation. My brain was obviously working at a slower rate due to the medication. It was a bizarre sensation, continuing a conversation that my friends had already finished.

Greg reduced the medication to 50mg daily, but I continued being confronted with images and flashbacks of various crime scenes. The question I could not answer was 'How can one human being do this to another?' I was also still suffering from lack of concentration and forgetfulness, leaving the oven on and the top of the gas stove alight.

Occasionally I had intrusive thoughts. Once I thought about getting my firearm from work and committing suicide. It would have been so easy. I knew the system and the police station process and procedures, and the location of the key to the firearm safe. I knew that if the supervisor and duty officer were occupied I would have a very good chance of obtaining these keys because of my rank as inspector. It was highly unlikely that a junior police officer would confront me about my actions.

My mind raced with the possibilities. The mental negotiation commenced: *Yes it's a possibility, but no you are not choosing this option,* I reminded myself. I chose to listen to the help I was being given instead.

I discussed this thought in a counselling session with Vera and later found that she had contacted my commander at St George to ensure I could not get access to my firearm. I was mortified. I hadn't wanted anyone to know about the suicidal thoughts. The reality was I was still not in a good place and I acknowledged Vera did the right thing.

By mid 2004, however, Greg described me as a 'walking time bomb wrapped in Christmas paper'. At every appointment I would walk in, smile and ask how he was. When he asked how I was feeling my standard non-thinking reply was, 'Good'. By the time the session was over it was quite clear I was *not* good. This was how I was going through life. I didn't want people to get close to my sorrow and distress because I was still concerned I could cause damage to others by telling them about it, as I thought I'd done with my first psychiatrist. (This vicarious traumatisation, as it is called, is a process of change that happens when you care about other people who have been hurt and feeling committed to or responsible for helping them.) I was continuing to keep my symptoms locked in a cupboard as I still couldn't deal with them. Instead, I adopted a Pollyanna approach to life. I might have accepted I had an illness but I was still fighting it. I showed concern for others in my life but couldn't show the same concern for myself. I wanted to feel better, but it wasn't happening fast enough for me.

I often thought about Solar Springs and felt fear about what had almost happened to me there. I felt afraid of that and wondered how I had got to that point. I knew how close I had come to choosing the peace of oblivion, and sometimes regretted having taken the harder path. Finally I felt positive: I was ill and had finally accepted that, and I now knew how other people in the same situation as mine might be feeling.

A woman at Jake's school had dark long hair and a skinny build. She reminded me of Michelle Miller, the prostitute killed by Nathan Kerr, and immediately I saw her as a walking corpse. When my mind became so confused, I remembered the calmness and serenity offered by that view of Morton National Park at Bundanoon. Then I felt guilty because I shouldn't have been thinking this way. Every time I closed my eyes my head felt as if it was spinning. I was still having counselling and psychotherapy sessions at least twice a week.

A dear friend of Rob's from the Special Air Service (SAS) based in Perth had recently come back from Afghanistan. He was very traumatised by things he had seen and been involved in, and I believed his situation was so much worse than ours.

I really felt for him. He told us he enjoyed so much coming over for dinner as he could relate to the way we were feeling. I was more than happy for him to come over any time if it helped him. We were all a little like zombies, all on our anti-depressant medication. Our SAS friend used to sit back and watch Rob and me get dinner, work around the house, or just generally chat to him. He later said the reason he so relished coming over was that our wacky emotional states made him feel good. At least we were helping someone, even if it was providing some amusement.

At this stage I had met a group of women through my daughter's dance lessons. During the one-hour class we would sit together and chat. I didn't tell them much about my background, only that I was a police officer on sick leave with PTSD. When Melanie first started the dance classes they were held on a day and time when I had a permanent counselling appointment. Rob told the women I had a weekly massage at that time and they were all envious. Later, when the class time changed and I took Melanie myself, I was too embarrassed to tell them the truth.

These women weren't aware of the incidents that had put me in this position and they had little idea what I was going through. I only gave minimal information to protect them and myself as I could still barely discuss the images in my head or the symptoms I was experiencing. I felt tainted by what I had seen and would look at these women and feel grateful they had never experienced the horrors I had: the broken bodies, the devastated families. I was glad they had not been exposed to this brutal side of life and they did not have to go through what I had suffered.

The antidepressant medication I was taking sometimes made me slow to absorb information. I found these women very tolerant when I continued with a conversation after they had finished it. They did not judge me and never commented about my strange behaviour. I consider myself fortunate that I am still associated with these wonderful women.

My family continued to have difficulty supporting me emotionally for a number of reasons and I had never asked for any support. When I finally succumbed to my symptoms and took sick leave, I was too proud to ask them for help and I did not want to be a burden to anyone. I was the person my family came to when they need to talk through something and I was concerned that I might traumatise them by detailing the situations in which I had been involved.

Recently I discussed this with a family member, whose response I believe applies to work colleagues and family alike. I was told that this person did not understand PTSD, what had caused it, what its associated symptoms are. A former work colleague told a friend flatly, 'I just don't get PTSD!'

I now know how to answer this. It is not necessary to have endured PTSD to understand what it is. Do your own research into the symptoms your loved one or colleague is displaying, either on the internet or by talking to a health professional. The best thing you can do is be there for the PTSD sufferer. Let them know you support them, listen without being judgmental, show them you care and can be called on at any time. At the very least an occasional phone call to your friend or family member will work wonders.

I certainly remember those who made the effort and thank them. What they did made a world of difference to me.

The end is also the beginning

It is only through acceptance that one may find peace.

Former hostage negotiator Nicole, 2013

The police rehabilitation officer called me several times, asking whether I was returning to work. I had asked Greg how long it would take for my brain to start functioning normally again. When would the forgetfulness disappear – in twelve months, five years, fifteen years? I might well have been asking 'How long is a piece of string?' I was still leaving home appliances on, forgetting to lock up the house when I went out and even neglecting basic hygiene. I had an MRI of the brain to ensure there were no organic problems. No, it was quite simply PTSD.

Towards the end of 2004 I had to accept I was not returning to work and submitted a medical discharge. I had already been advised that my command was going to submit one if I didn't, as they needed to readvertise and fill my position. I knew my career as a police officer was over.

I was devastated by this. I was so proud of what I had achieved. I'd had the opportunity to work at some of the most interesting and highly intensive areas in policing. I never once shirked responsibility and always gave every situation my best effort. I had received numerous letters of appreciation from members of the public and other senior police officers, as well as awards and commendations. In 2003 I had been awarded the National Medal for over fifteen years of diligent service. In 2004 I was awarded the NSW Police Medal for ten years of ethical and diligent service, including the first clasp, as recognition for an additional five years. I did not want to leave. I still had things I wanted to achieve.

The horrendous flashbacks of the homicide scenes I had attended continued to plague me. In particular, whenever Rob was angry I would get a flashback of the bruised face of Donna Wheeler. Rob had never hit me but my PTSD-induced fears made me worry that being a strong man he might strike me in anger. Then I could be dead just like Donna Wheeler. My children would no longer have a mother. This continued to play on my mind and whenever Rob became agitated I grew edgier.

By early 2005 I couldn't cope any longer. It was a vicious cycle, my symptoms, my irritability, forgetfulness, and lack of concentration were affecting Rob's stress levels, and his agitation and anger were affecting mine. We had been undergoing marriage counselling for eighteen months but I couldn't manage it any more. I was at the point where I couldn't handle

Rob's anger and the thought of dying due to a punch to the face. I could no longer stay in the marriage for the sake of the children. I knew if I were to continue as a mother and look after my children I needed to start looking after myself as a priority.

In February 2005 our marriage was over. We both agreed to end the marriage before we ended up hating each other. It was a huge weight off our shoulders for both of us.

We sat down and told the children. Jake was six and a half years old and Melanie was three and a half. I feel Jake accepted what was happening at that time due to all the arguing he had witnessed. Melanie just followed her big brother; she was too young to understand what was going on.

Rob and I both put the children first; they had not asked to be in this situation. I took on a major mortgage to buy the family home from Rob. I wanted to try and minimise the disruption for the children, to maintain some stability for them. Rob stayed in the house until April, when he moved into his own home only ten minutes' drive away. We were both off work, both mentally ill, so there was no custody dispute over the children. Without the need for solicitors we decided on a shared custody arrangement that remains in place today.

I would be lying if I said things were easy after our marriage ended. I was a single mother with two small children and struggling with PTSD. It was a very difficult time and I knew if I didn't look after myself I would never get better. Then I had the good fortune to discover a book called *Crime Scene* by Esther McKay, a former forensic investigator with the NSW Police. It was her account of working as a forensic investigator and her subsequent breakdown after developing post-traumatic stress disorder.

This was the first time I had been able to relate to another person's thoughts, symptoms and feelings about PTSD. I no longer felt so alienated and isolated. I was no longer the only person feeling like this. The book, in effect, normalised what I was going through.

My breathing exercises continued, together with my daily quiet time sessions and ongoing psychotherapy. The antidepressant medication I continued to take numbed my emotions, but it did not help improve my memory or many other symptoms, including the terrible flashbacks and mood swings.

In August 2005 Greg conducted a study of 'putative cerebellum exercises' involving fourteen of his patients (see Appendix). The cerebellum, sometimes called the miniature brain, is a separate structure attached to the bottom of the brain. It has always been known as critical for balance and motor function and more recent research has revealed that, as well as having an important cognitive function, it may have an impact on emotional memory.

I was prepared to try anything to relieve my symptoms so I agreed to take part. I was given various simple exercises and instructions on how to do them. The goal was to carry out a simple balance exercise regularly, to make the cerebellum work harder. We would take a 'Black Box' approach – in between the 'exercises' and the 'result' is what we might call the Black Box, for arguments sake. Whilst we do not know what was occurring in the Black Box, research has indicated that, based on PTSD and other conditions, including Attention Deficit Hyperactivity Disorder (ADHD) where these types of exercises have been used, that these exercises may have an effect on the cerebellum and its impact on emotional memory. This is yet to be proven and thoroughly tested, I can only provide my experience and the effect these exercises had on me. The science behind this is a matter for discussion for experts, not for this book; I will focus on what occurred next in my recovery.

I went home that afternoon feeling optimistic for the first time in ages. I wanted to get better and, hopefully, discontinue the antidepressant medication. However, it was made very clear to me that these exercises only constituted part of my therapy. I would continue to receive the usual treatments for PTSD, including psychotherapy and/or cognitive behavioural therapy and medication.

I was told to do these exercises twice a day for only five minutes each time. Strict adherence to this regime was critical to success. The first exercise involved balancing on one foot with my eyes closed. I was to keep my other foot close to the ground in case I felt unsteady or about to overbalance. If I did feel as if I was about to fall, I should use my other foot to steady myself, rather than my hands. I was also allowed to change feet if my leg started to ache.

I used the microwave timer in the kitchen and did the exercise morning and night. I was told that if it was difficult, then it was likely my cerebellum was working very hard to regain that balance. After nearly three weeks, I was finally able to balance for five minutes on one foot with my eyes closed. I noticed I was starting to feel calmer around the children. I was still irritable but there was an underlying feeling of good, no longer the destructive feelings of anger. It was as though the veil of depression was lifting. My memory was still terrible, however, I was no longer feeling frustrated from the loss of my former capabilities. I was starting to accept my 'ditsy' state.

After I'd successfully completed the first exercise I was given the second one. This involved balancing on one foot with my eyes closed and my arms held out to the sides at shoulder level. Very slowly and keeping my arms straight, I was to bring my hands to the centre and touch my index fingers together. This movement was to be done no more than twice in the allocated five minutes.

I continued with more exercises, which involved the purchase of a wobble board/balance board and a set of juggling balls. First, I had to balance on the board with two feet and my eyes open. Then I added the extra task of throwing a juggling ball from one hand to the other at eye level. Next, I had to throw two juggling balls and finally three. Again, I did the exercises for only five minutes twice a day. I had to successfully complete the previous exercise before I started a new one.

I was amazed at the difference all this made to my symptoms. After three weeks I had permission to wean myself from the antidepressant medication.

By the end of August 2005, I had my first night out with some close girlfriends after over two years of withdrawal and avoidance of social situations. For the first time in years I was starting to remember what it was like to feel happy again.

The core group of patients, of which I was one, all started seeing results within one to three weeks of doing these exercises. I even began to sleep better and my feelings of anxiety lessened. At the end of August 2005, while driving to Coffs Harbour with my mother, I experienced a vision of an accident similar to an earlier intrusive thought. When I turned around to check on Melanie in the back seat, I imagined her head severed from her neck and blood pouring out. However, I did not get the same heightened feelings of panic and anxiety that I had experienced on the first occasion, nor did the feelings last as long. This was a major breakthrough for me.

I still have lots of terrible memories, but they are becoming more distant. I can now control the thoughts; they do not control me. People with PTSD continue to relive horrific situations, but once I started the exercises my recollections became less immediate. People who do not have PTSD may wonder why someone cannot 'let go' of a horrific experience, however, PTSD is about having a recurrent, contemporary experience. Sufferers constantly relive the experience and thus react as though the horror had just been seen or felt for the first time.

I still live with PTSD, but I have learned to recognise what triggers an escalation in my symptoms. Knowledge is power. This allows me to better manage myself and use the various techniques I have learned. I have found that when I am most stressed my balance is not good. I have also established that whilst the putative cerebellum exercises do not resolve PTSD they definitely assist in the reduction of some of my symptoms.

I am still an overprotective mother. I once photographed my son before he went out with a friend and his friend's father. Not unusual you may think, but my reason for taking the photograph was in case Jake became lost or kidnapped, so I had the best possible evidence of what he looked like and clothes he was wearing at the time. I no longer do this. Fortunately my mental health is improving, slowly but surely.

Numerous parents tell me they also have fears in relation to their children. An expert told me that, yes, all parents have fears; the difference for those with my traumatic background is that we have the gallery of images to add an extra dimension to these fears.

I am very fortunate to be surrounded by a supportive group of friends and family members. If my symptoms escalate, for example, if I start to become very busy to the point of being hyperactive, one of them will soon point that out to me. I can then identify the stressor and work on it. I also have no problem ringing a friend and saying, 'Hey, I'm having a shocker, have you got a minute?' something I rarely did before the treatment. I can even tell my children I need time out, especially when I am irritable, and disappear to the bedroom for half an hour. They accept this and understand that it assists me.

I still suffer badly with my memory and concentration. If someone waved at me and I didn't acknowledge them I wasn't being rude, I just didn't recognise them. To combat that, I now just smile and nod at everyone I see. I still have symptoms of hyperarousal – feeling tense, having an exaggerated 'startle response', and remaining in the 'flight or fight' mode, being hypervigilant and suffering fatigue – although not to the extent that I suffered them in the past. I still jump at loud noises but I'm no longer diving to the floor or checking for intruders.

I have had only one major setback that required me to go back on the antidepressant medication for a period of time. This was caused by the stress of filing a duty of care civil suit against the NSW Police Force. After almost four years of highly stressful negotiation, we settled out of court. Now the case is over I can continue in my recovery.

CHAPTER

23

PTSD and what can be done

Policing is sometimes to referred to as a contact sport. It is an occupation that carries risks to both physical and emotional health. The issue is when it is known how risk can be minimised, but the appropriate steps are not put in place. Since I succumbed to PTSD a series of measures have been adopted, including additional psychological and welfare checks on police in the areas I worked. The real concern, however, is the constant exposure to traumatic situations. I believe there is scope for change in this area that would benefit the NSW Police Force and its officers.

Psychiatrist Dr Greg Wilkins, who has been treating NSW police officers for over twenty-five years, has said, 'If the police serviced their cars the same way they service their personnel, it would mean removing all warning lights, oil and water gauges from the dashboard, welding down the bonnet, and as soon as the vehicle stops going or starts blowing smoke, discard the vehicle and get a new one!'

Professor Alexander McFarlane, a leading world expert in PTSD and the head of the University of Adelaide Centre for Traumatic Stress Studies, says the more people are exposed to trauma on a regular basis, such as soldiers, police or paramedics, the more their brain changes and the body's stress system becomes more sensitive. 'The idea is that people get tougher and get used to things and the effects of stress go away,' he states. 'The fascinating thing is that the body actually does keep score and so next time around you are so much more vulnerable.'

Early intervention is crucial in treating PTSD, and the best person to detect signs of potential psychological dysfunction is a supervisor or family member. One of the first things a PTSD-affected person loses is the ability to monitor their own emotional state and track their internalised world.

This may explain why I never believed I had a problem. If I had, I could have sought assistance many years earlier and perhaps my symptoms would not have been so severe. Perhaps I could have taken time out before the next trauma exposure.

A joint paper by Professor Alexander McFarlane and Professor Richard Bryant (University of NSW), 'Post-traumatic stress disorder in occupational setting: anticipating and managing the risk', states that:

> ...it can be useful if supervisors can detect signs that may indicate an individual is experiencing some PTSD reactions. The negative impact of traumatic events can manifest in a variety of indirect ways which employers should be alert to.

- Increased alcohol use
- Interpersonal and/or family conflict
- Social withdrawal
- Depression

- Somatic distress (physical pain and discomfort)
- Performance deterioration

In June 2011, anonymous survey results were published as a result of a review of injury management practices in the NSW Police Force. Taking into account the signs listed by professors McFarlane and Bryant, it is interesting to note the different perceptions of the police hierarchy and the psychologically injured worker. Managers, duty officers and commanders expressed frustration that psychological injury claims were accepted as a result of workplace conflict or conduct issues. No consideration was given that workplace conflict and conduct issues could possibly stem from a psychological injury.

Injured workers expressed frustration at the lack of support from their commanders and management, believing there needs to be a change in culture and perception of injured officers. One person surveyed referred to 'comments by commander that they thought my injury was not genuine'.

This survey was initiated seven years after I was diagnosed with PTSD, but these were the very same attitudes I encountered with my own commander and a duty officer when I went off on sick leave.

As a result of this review the NSW Police Force introduced the Workforce Improvement Plan, a major part of which advocated improved education and awareness in all police, combined with training in injury management and interpersonal communication skills for supervisors and senior management. Another notable recommendation was increasing leadership development to all ranks. If these recommendations are properly carried out they will constitute an important and well overdue change in the current culture. The recommendations must be implemented to have an effect.

The Australian Army has taken a similar approach. Retired General Peter Cosgrove has admitted his former scepticism about psychological health programs and adds, 'I have changed my mind, because what the evidence shows is the earlier the intervention and support given to any soldier diagnosed with a psychological problem, the better the chance they have to minimise its effects ... The key is the availability of, and access to, experts in post-traumatic stress' (*Newcastle Herald*, 24 April 2013).

Early intervention can involve anything and everything, including

- Supervisors tracking their individual team members' trauma load
- Supervisors identifying potential psychologically affected officers
- Discreet one-on-one conversations between the injured officer and an appropriate supervisor with follow up and support
- Removal or respite from frontline duties or from further exposure for a specific period
- Referral to mental-health professionals who have credibility and experience in PTSD
- The prescription of appropriate medication if required

The credibility of both supervisors and mental-health professionals is paramount, otherwise the psychologically affected officer will never declare his or her concerns. I know of incidents within the NSW Police Wellcheck program where officers have been sent for health checks to junior psychologists who have little or no experience with PTSD. Sometimes they have been sent to a different psychologist each time so no continuity or significant building of rapport was possible.

While there is much research to support early intervention, the situation of the psychologically injured worker who has seen horror or been continually exposed to trauma also needs to be considered. It may be impossible to minimise the effects of PTSD for someone in this situation. It is these emergency and defence-force personnel that I especially feel for. I have been there, as have close friends of mine.

The best advice I can offer to fellow sufferers is this. Firstly, psychoeducation is critical. Gather knowledge about your condition, whether it's PTSD or another ailment. Ask your mental-health professional for information about your illness, and speak to others who have been in a similar position. They understand! My research helped me gain insight into my condition, and into why I was acting in a particular way. It served to make me feel less alienated and gave me a focus on how I could help myself.

Secondly, accept that you have a problem. With acceptance comes the ability to receive the right treatment. You will no longer struggle to understand why you are behaving in an unusual way. You will have the tools to help you manage your condition, even though there will still be good and bad days. Let your family in, and they will help you. You need support, and once you accept this you will better manage your symptoms.

You can't stop the waves, but you can learn to surf.
Joseph Goldstein

I recall a day in 2012 where I was surfing beyond the break. I was still a novice board rider but I caught an amazing wave. I stood up and rode this green unbroken wave for what seemed like forever. It felt as if I almost made it onto the shore before it broke.

It was exhilarating. Grinning from ear to ear, I paddled back out to where the seasoned surfers were all waiting for a wave. A few of them gave me a smile and a couple made comment on the 'good wave', or 'good ride' I had. I laughed, saying, 'I finally felt like a real surfer.'

After years of struggling in the surf, trying to swim against the current and being smashed by the waves I no longer feel as if my head is underwater and I am gasping for breath. I am finally enjoying the ride and I am confident of the journey ahead.

It has been a very difficult journey and there have been setbacks, but each day life gets better.

APPENDIX

The use of Putative Cerebellum Exercises to Control and Relieve Symptoms of PTSD

by Greg Wilkins

Post-traumatic Stress Disorder (PTSD) is a disabling disorder that affects approximately 8% of the population at some point in their life. The disorder is associated with significant morbidity and functional impairment. The pathophysiology of PTSD involves a complex interaction between trauma-related factors and the neurobiological and psychosocial influences that determine individual differences in resilience and vulnerability[1].

Patients who present with PTSD exhibit a change in their cognitive function which manifests as specific problems with attention shifting, attention splitting, following instructions, short-term memory, poor impulse control, and a distorted sense of linear time.

In the early 1990s, Prof McFarlane[2] referred to PTSD as sharing some of the cardinal features of Attention

Deficit Hyperactivity Disorder (ADHD). Several programs report improvement in cognitive function of patients with ADHD[3] using physical exercise techniques believed to stimulate the cerebellum. They also report improvement in several other features of patients with ADHD, i.e., impulse control, short-term memory, sense of time, connectedness to others and communication ability. While the neurophysiological processes underlying these benefits are unclear, the empirical evidence prompted us to examine the benefits of such exercises on PTSD.

Two patients with (PTSD) are presented who used 'cerebellar-stimulating' exercises as means of managing their PTSD symptoms.

A thirty-five-year-old female patient who had been exposed to multiple traumas over many years presented with longstanding symptoms of PTSD. She had participated in several types of therapy including medication and cognitive behavioural therapy (flooding, cognitive reframing) with minimal impact on her symptoms. Specifically she described avoidance, hyperarousal, preservative thoughts reliving specific traumas, physical symptoms of anxiety, flashbacks, intrusive thoughts, nightmares, poor sleep, emotional numbing, a distorted sense of linear time, poor short-term memory, poor concentration, poor planning and execution of tasks, difficulty following conversations and feelings of depersonalisation.

She was introduced to a novel physical exercise designed to stimulate her cerebellar function. The patient stood and balanced on a wobble board while juggling two balls. This exercise was performed for five minutes twice daily.

The patient reported a marked improvement in all aspects of her symptoms within the first two weeks of commencing this exercise regime. Of note was a marked shift in her ability to recall details of her various traumas, and to talk about them without developing dissociation and anxiety seen prior to commencing the exercise. She stopped the exercises after twelve weeks. Three months after ceasing the exercises she had maintained her recovery. She has not received other treatment since the time of commencing the exercises and she has remained well. Her initial PTSD Checklist – Civilian score was 78 and fell to 25 after performing the exercise[4].

The second patient was a twenty-four-year-old male who had suffered a single horrific incident several months prior to presenting in which he had sustained several physical injuries and seen several close colleagues seriously injured. He described persistent symptoms of hyperarousal, re-experiencing specific sounds and pictures of the trauma, physical symptoms of anxiety, intrusive thoughts, nightmares, poor sleep, emotional numbing, social withdrawal to the point of not being able to leave his house, a distorted sense of linear time, poor short-term memory, poor concentration, poor task completion, unable to participate in conversations other than brief and superficial interactions with his partner and a feeling of depersonalisation.

He was diagnosed as suffering with acute PTSD. He was introduced to the putative cerebellar exercise. He was asked to stand on one leg and close his eyes until he became unstable when he would either open his eyes or lower his leg to regain his stability. Once stable he would repeat the exercise and this continued for five minutes twice daily. His initial PTSD Checklist – Civilian score was 72 and fell to 42 after performing the exercise.

He continued the exercise for six weeks and reported a marked improvement, which continued for further six weeks after ceasing the exercise. He described a calming effect and was also able to give a detailed account of the trauma without the recurrence of his symptoms. He was able to feel the anger and fear without re-experiencing the actual trauma as he had invariably done prior to commencing the exercises.

Since these exercises involved balance and postural control, they stimulate the cerebellum. The role of the cerebellum in cognitive function has come under increasing scrutiny. In an examination of carefully matched cohort of children who had experienced significant psychological or emotional trauma, De Bellis demonstrated that the cerebellum of the traumatised subjects was significantly reduced in volume from that of the controls[5]. The traumatised subjects were also likely to suffer from an ADHD-like syndrome.

A group of fourteen patients suffering with PTSD have been assessed and treated with the conventional treatment for PTSD and the putative cerebellar exercise. The duration of treatment ranges from four to twelve weeks. The results confirm a benefit in the relief of PTSD symptoms as indicated by the PCL-C scores (see figure 1).

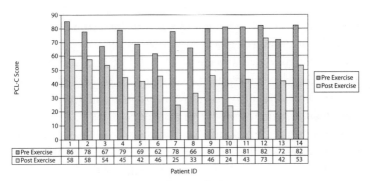

Patient ID	1	2	3	4	5	6	7	8	9	10	11	12	13	14
Pre Exercise	86	78	67	79	69	62	78	66	80	81	81	82	72	82
Post Exercise	58	58	54	45	42	46	25	33	46	24	43	73	42	53

Figure 1

McFarlane[6] has proposed a neural network model of PTSD, which is relevant for our current understanding:

in PTSD repetition instigates the mechanisms of iterative learning, top-down activation and pruning. The

*development of the symptoms of PTSD being explained
by current knowledge about modelling disturbances of
parallel distributed processing. The noradrenergic neu-
rones play a central role in co-ordinating the interaction
of multiple cortical regions, which is an essential aspect of
parallel distributed processing. Disturbances of this system
in PTSD are likely to manifest as a dysfunctional modula-
tion of working memory and involuntary traumatic recollection. Modifications of neural networks have a secondary
effect of kindling in the hippocampus that further mod-
erates the individual's sensitivity to a range of stressors.
Therefore, a neural network model of PTSD provides a
method for conceptualising the onset of PTSD symptoms
and their subsequent modification with the passage of time.*

Consistent with this model is that the cerebellum has been
referred to as *an adaptive controller*[7], i.e., *a system having
the capability to adjust or optimise its own parameters automatically*. One of the likely functions of the cerebellum is to
provide the 'timing or clock' by which neural networks are set
and regulated, timed and co-ordinated. In PTSD and ADHD,
symptoms may come about as a result of some flaw in this
'clock'. This disruption or flaw would account for many of
the cardinal symptoms of both disorders.

The dramatic reduction in symptoms in this group of
patients suggests that this mode of treatment warrants sys-
tematic investigation. If the efficacy is indeed established, the
underlying neurobiological processes can be investigated.

The current hypothesis is that the exercise(s), which is (are)
relatively complex and require considerable processing of
data by the cerebellar, may invoke some restoration / correc-
tion of *the adaptive controller*, i.e., cerebellar function.

Footnotes

1. Connor KM., MD. and Marian I. Butterfield, MD., M.P.H. Focus *Posttraumatic Stress Disorder REVIEW* 1:247–262 (2003) © 2003 American Psychiatric Association

2. McFarlane AC., Weber DL. and Clark CR., *Abnormal stimulus processing in posttraumatic stress disorder.,* Biological Psychiatry. 34(5):311–20, 1 September 1993

3. The DORE Program, Mind Gym

4. DeBellis M., *Developmental Traumatology: Neurobiological Development of Maltreated Children with PTSD.* Paper presented at the Royal Australian and New Zealand College of Psychiatrist on 24 May 2005, Sydney, Australia

5. Weathers F., Litz, Huska & Keane, *Posttraumatic Stress Disorder Symptom Checklist – Civilian Version (PCL_C for DSM-IV),* National Centre for PTSD (11/1/1994)

6. McFarlane AC., Yehuda R. and Clark CR., *Biologic models of traumatic memories and post-traumatic stress disorder. The role of neural networks.* Psychiatric Clinics of North America. 25(2): 253–70, v, June 2002

7. Barlow, John S., in 'The Cerebellum and Adaptive Control', Chapter 17, pp273, *The Cerebellum as an Adaptive Controller,* pub Cambridge University Press, 2002

SOURCES

This book is drawn from my memory of various incidents with help from my duty books, police incident reports, briefs of evidence — including statements and transcripts of interviews — NSW police negotiator reports and course notes, fellow investigators, negotiators and tactical police, the Australian Police Journal, court reports, and my diaries. In addition I acknowledge specific assistance in the listed chapters.

Chapter 2 *Sydney Morning Herald* article dated 23 June 1989. 'Sweethearts at 6am: Shots and a man dies'.

Chapter 3 The National Guidelines for the Deployment of Police in High Risk Situations – Australasian Centre for Policing Research. Police Commissioners' Policy Advisory Group, 1992.

State Protection Group, Negotiation Unit, Lecture notes

Tactical Advice: thanks to Rob, former Senior Instructor Level 3 and Tactical Team Leader.

State Protection Support Unit Course report 1994

Chapter 5 Recollections from Rob concerning incident at Burwood.

Chapter 6 R v De Gruchy [2000] NSWCCA 51 (2 March 2000)

Chapter 7 R v Mailes [2003] NSWSC 707 (1 August 2003)

Chapter 9 R v Martin and Cushman [1999] NSWSC 1048 (14 September 1999)

Chapter 10 NSW Police Service Weekly Vol 8 No 3, 22 January, 1996 p8

Chapter 13 Regina v Offer [2000] NSWSC 839 (25 August 2000)

R v Offer [2002] NSWCCA 341 (20 August 2002)

Australian Police Journal September 2003, Vol 57 No 3 article 'Unholy Offerings' by Senior Constable David Gardner

Chapter 15 R v Bond [2000] NSWSC 1059 (7 December 2000)

http://www.abc.net.au/news/2005-03-14/inmate-dies-at-lithgow-jail/1532770

Chapter 16 R v Kerr [2002] NSWSC 309 (12 April 2002)

Chapter 22 McKay, Esther. *Crime Scene*. Penguin Group (Australia), 2005.

Advice from Dr Greg Wilkins concerning Cerebellum exercises

Chapter 23 Henderson, Michelle. 'Traumatic events affect bodies years later.' NSW Police News, Vol 92 No 8 August 2012. p32.

McFarlane, Alexander C and Bryant, Richard A. "Post-traumatic stress disorder in occupational settings: anticipating and managing the risk." Occupational Medicine 2007; 57:404-410.

NSW Police Force, Review of Injury Management Practices – June 2011.

RESOURCES

For suicide and crisis support Lifeline 13 11 14 or Beyond Blue 1300 22 4636 www.beyondblue.org.au

For support and information about depression and anxiety Black Dog Institute www.blackdoginstitute.org.au

For information about symptoms, treatment and prevention of depression and bipolar disorder — SANE Australia Helpline 1800 187263 www.sane.org

For information about mental illness, treatments and where to go for support

Alcoholics Anonymous Australia 1300 222222 www.aa.org.au

I would also advise informing your family doctor and perhaps giving them information from the following websites so that they understand more about PTSD — www.som.uq.edu.au/ptsd - University of Queensland School of Medicine has developed the Posttraumatic Stress Disorder (PTSD) evidence based information resource and www.acpmh.unimelb.edu.au - Australian Centre for Posttraumatic Mental Health

ACKNOWLEDGEMENTS

Under Siege has been five years in the making and I can honestly say it was not a cathartic experience. To try and give the reader the best and most accurate description of what I was seeing and how I was feeling at the time, I needed to relive those situations. This aggravated my symptoms and sent me on a downward spiral a number of times, but the message about PTSD I was trying to convey was too important to cease writing. Now the book is complete, I would like to express my sincere appreciation to a number of people who supported me, listened to me, gave me advice, and had faith in me.

Dr Greg Wilkins. I cannot thank you enough for all your help over the years. For your wisdom, for getting me through some very difficult times, for helping rebuild confidence in myself again. Thank you also for all your advice and guidance with the book; to help explain PTSD symptoms to the reader. Thank you also for those wonderful cerebellum exercises.

Vera Auerbach, you were the first person I felt comfortable enough with to talk to about my symptoms. Your diagnosis of PTSD was the start of my recovery. I thank you for your wonderful guidance through some very dark times.

Karen Davis (author of *Sinister Intent* and one of my dearest friends). Thank you for all your writing advice, editing, support, and having faith in me that I could do it also. Most of all, thank you for all our wonderful years of friendship — twenty seven in fact ;)

Nicole Bramah, another of my dearest friends. Thank you for all your support and for just being there, not only through my years of writing. Thank you also for editing and being my sounding board on all aspects of negotiation. You are truly the queen.

Michelle Walker (Proco), my dearest school friend. You were always there if I needed you, although I could never tell you how bad it became until much later. You are an incredible woman and I feel privileged to call you my friend.

Mum and Dad — both incredibly intelligent people and avid readers — thank you, not only for the brilliant editing, but for all your love and support over the years.

Dad and Michelle, thank you for making me feel so at home and providing me with an escape in sunny Cairns when I need recovery time :)

Michelle Menzies, thank you also for all the support you have given to me over the last few years and the clarification of the mediation process.

Sharon, my sister, thank you for being there, for checking on me when you knew my breathing was shallow from associated anxiety issues and other PTSD symptoms, or when I was having the odd breakdown. I have shared many of my most memorable moments with you. Love you sis.

Marilyn Inglis, thank you so much for taking the time out to edit my book and give me an unbiased view. It is very much appreciated.

Nicola O'Shea, I am so grateful for the structural work you did on my chronological police report. You provided amazing insight and turned my manuscript into a document that provided the right themes, emotion and interest. A document I was proud to show to my agent.

Selwa Anthony, my literary agent. I am still in shock that you took me on and made my wish come true. Thank you so much for having faith in me. Thank you for all your support, advice and guidance in a world I know nothing about. You are truly the doyenne of the publishing world.

To the team at Harlequin, my publishers. I still feel overwhelmed by all the support and the belief you have in me. Thank you for making me feel so welcome. You are all truly amazing. I particularly want to mention Michelle, Sue, Cristina, Jo and the wonderfully talented Adam. Jo Mackay, you are the most beautiful person, it has been lovely working so closely with you.

Jacqueline Kent, I feel privileged that someone as talented as you was interested in editing my book. Thank you so much not only for the work you did but for taking the time to learn where I was coming from.

Mark Whittaker, journalist. Thank you so much for the sensitivity you showed in the article 'Back from the Brink', it was a wonderful story. Thank you also for taking the time to edit some of my first chapters. I'm doing my best not to use too many capitals anymore ;)

My ex husband 'Rob', tactical operative extraordinaire. You lived this with me. You know the hell we went through. Thank you so much for your support and for all the tactical advice and guidance for the book.

Angelo Memmolo — my favourite and best looking work partner ever :) Thank you so much for all your support over the years, and input into the 'Psychopath' chapter. You were one who rang to genuinely see how I was going. Thank you so much for that.

Andrew Marks — Marksy, thank you for all your support during my time at St George LAC. Thank you also for the genuine phone calls asking after my health. I truly appreciate that.

Russell Oxford, thank you so much for the help provided in the 'Which Brother?' chapter. You, alongside others I have mentioned in my book including Wayne Hayes and Wayne Gordon are some of the most amazing investigators I worked with.

My surfing group, the motorcyclists I ride with, my former Friday morning ladies netball comp, and my wonderful gal pals – thanks for keeping me sane during the writing of my book.

Lastly and most importantly, to my two gorgeous children. I am so amazed at how wonderful you both are, even being subject to a household with two parents with PTSD and our marriage breakdown. You are both so intelligent, caring and strong. One day when you read this book, when you are older ;), I hope it can bring you some understanding of what we were all going through. Thank you for the hugs when I needed them most and the help around the house. Thank you for being understanding when I needed my half hour time outs. I am in awe of you both. Much love to you.